GRAND MAL

by

Joshua Holmes

JAHbookdesign | York, PA

AUTHOR'S NOTE

Just a quick note to my readers: I loosely based this novella on my collegiate experience and the master's program from which I graduated. While I visited several of the described places and participated in several of the classes, the characters are fictional and the expressed philosophies and worldviews aren't necessarily all mine. For the most part, this is fictional.

That said, the seizures I describe and the feelings and scenarios associated with them are real. I have to cope with them regularly, and I wanted my reader to better understand what persons with epilepsy deal with, and ultimately to see what we are capable of.

I went back and forth about the main character's name, as it is basically me with the name 'Chris.' Although I finally went with the aforementioned name, it is my hope that the cast of characters and scenes and unbeatable setting make up for anything lackluster in the name of Chris. Thanks for your support.

– Josh

GRAND MAL

A NOVELLA

JOSHUA HOLMES

PART ONE:

YEAR ONE, SUMMER SEMESTER, SEASONS PAST

THE BUS stop is about ten feet away, near a large ditch, and I plan to sit on a bench until the bus arrives. I have a spot on the bench with my name on it. Chris is my name, and I intend to enjoy a grand summer day, a day with no painful events. The possibility is about to turn unlikely.

I am walking, looking at the golf course just across the way. The green is beautiful, the light turf against the dark rough a vivid landscape, the trees an added accent. The sun is high above in a cloudless sky, and people are riding around in golf carts with their clubs in the back rack. I am walking in a haze. Not a dark haze; a bright haze, if anything. I see the beauty, but I also see more. I see through it, feel a deeper sense of my surroundings. The sense is in my eyes, and in the back of my mouth, an unwanted view and a foul taste. I hope the deeper sense goes away.

I have been walking in this haze for most of the day. I have been living life as I normally would, but I have been carrying a heavy burden, the burden of disastrous possibilities. The possibilities of what may result from these strange sensations, this haze. I just have a small hope my day will continue without interruption.

The sense stays, however, and all of the sudden, it happens. The next thing I know, my body is twisting. My head slowly turns in the right direction, and it continues until my right shoulder rotates in the same direction. My chest is next, and, before I know it, I am falling. A long, hard fall.

I hope someone is near the bus stop, but it doesn't appear there is. If someone was there, I could say, "I'm not feeling good, I need help." Or something along those lines. To my chagrin, however, I don't get the opportunity.

Shortly after, I am on the ground, a road I think. Shaking. Not the kind of shaking most people experience when they are cold or when they have seen something frightening. I mean uncontrollable physical shaking.

I slide towards the ditch that has no business being there. It is right against the pavement. My face digs into the surface. I have faced many surfaces, both indoors and outdoors, yet I still haven't grown accustomed to the burn from my chin rubbing against gravel as black as night, or my forehead attaching itself like a stray weed with strong roots.

GRAND MAL

Strangely enough, I feel no pain when my body suffers. I know it will be bad when I get myself under control. When that happens, if it ever happens, my facial wounds will scream with intensity unlike any other; and my head will pound like a massive wave capsizing a sleepy town. Akin to a punctured ship, my body gradually sinks to the ground.

Upon impact, I bounce off the ground, and roll downward. I am aware of this, because I feel as if I am sliding on an angle. I try to stop rolling, but I am unsuccessful in my attempts. I try to position my body so I won't hit a solid protrusion, whatever it might be.

Soon, though, I am in a deep ditch with no enclaves or rocks to grab onto. Despite my best efforts to avoid injury, I hit something hard, as if I am a swimmer entangled in coral. The walls are too steep. I grapple, but the pebbles just loosen and crumble under my fingertips. I grapple and grapple some more, but the smaller stones start to slide down the wall. I stop momentarily, physically spent. Inside me though, a subconscious force urges me to keep trying. I subconsciously listen.

I hear a voice above me. It says, "I think he fell in the ditch. Over here."

"Yeah, he did," another voice sounds. "I see some foot tracks." Had I seen through some people? I am almost certain no one was around me.

"I'm gonna go check if he's alright."

It feels as if I have been in this ditch for quite some time now. I am sweating profusely, my shirt wet. Maybe it is starting to rain. I don't know. I think I'm starting to go delirious. I look up and ask for this to be over. It's wishful thinking.

The shadows along the walls are lengthy and grey. It was sunny earlier, I know, but there has been a lapse of light since I fell. Darkness covers me now. Gloom, too. Perhaps my current situation has exacerbated my perceptions. It's hard to say.

I groan, struggling to pull myself upright. I try to prop myself up against the dirt wall next to the bench near the bus stop, but I fail. When I hit the bottom of the ditch, most of my body stopped working.

The voices I heard earlier now have faces. Above me, I see two sets of eyes. They all feel sinister. Their stare is penetrating. I see two evil open mouths gawking. They are close to invading my space; an unwanted space, yet my own. I am close to feeling violated. I already have to fight the surface, my own dead body. Now I might have to fight for an open area with no one near.

At one point, I could have hollered for help. Not anymore. When I fell, that was the moment my ability to speak escaped me. I can't even spit out the granules of dirt that have taken my teeth and gum line captive. This is the way it is every time. Inside my throat I am screaming, but no sound escapes my lips. *Just stay away*, I think. *Leave me alone!*

Rarely, though, do people opt to leave me be. The next thing I know, I see an extended arm, and a pointing finger above me. "Should we call the police?"

"Probably. Do you have a cell?" *Shoot!* I think.

• • •

GRAND MAL

I'VE LEARNED to make those who discover me feel better through witticism. If I can laugh about my body contortions, my tremors, my laborious heaving, it appears to make others consider my abnormalities unimportant and something not worth getting upset over. I like it this way, yet I'll never know what they truly feel.

"So, I had the shakes, huh?" I question with a smile.

My friend Michael says, "Yeah Chris. Probably the worst in a while." He acts as if it's no big deal, the response I always hope for. "It's over though. Back to the good life?"

I look at him. He still has a baby face, as round as when I first met him. He has red hair, grizzle on his cheeks, now, and a red goatee. He is well built, also more muscular than I am. He is more outgoing, and quicker to hang with everyone, which explains his reputation as a fun loving guy.

He wasn't always the social butterfly though, the initiator of conversation. In fact, while he was the first to brave my malady, and step out and protect me during a seizure when we were in grade school, he was quite apprehensive to talk. He grew up in a conservative, religious home where it was evil to speak unless spoken to, to have colored hair, tattoos, or piercings for that matter. This mentality branched out into every other area of his life, ultimately forcing him to refrain from any commentary. But he wanted to speak, and eventually became sick of the legalism. He grew weary of hearing "or else you are going to hell."

Whenever Michael did something a little rebellious and heard the threat as a teen, he would say, "Whatever. Back to the good life."

So, kind of joking, I say, "Right. Back to the good life." Truthfully, though, my brain is in a state of turmoil, incredible tides of pain lap on my head of sand.

Michael and I live in a two-room apartment. We split a bathroom, share a small but suitable kitchen, and often recline on the couches in our condensed living room. We agreed I could decorate the living room with my artwork, and he could practice his culinary skills any way he wished in the kitchen. The agreement seems to have worked thus far.

In a short-sleeved Polo shirt and long Cargo shorts, he is standing by the window, a floor to ceiling frame of glass through which you can see the bus stop. "I saw you fall down there," he says, his one hand rubbing his goatee, his other hand in his pocket. "They really need to fill in that ditch."

Michael and I have been friends for years, since adolescence. When we finished high school, we both decided to go to Penn State University, so we wouldn't have to face the postsecondary academic world alone. It has turned out to be a good decision, because, despite the size of this university, we never felt too overwhelmed, and at this point, at ages twenty-five and twenty-six, we find it far from daunting.

I walk over to the window. It is getting dark outside. "Yeah." I say, "That's for sure."

• • •

STILL AT the window, I think of one thing I initially had difficulty with. My ability to communicate with my professors. I found the task irritating, because, in general, my academic success in the Counselor Education program ultimately hinges on the opinions of my superiors. This might be a surprise, but, in the past, I have had several run-ins with one professor. Mrs. Patterson. At times, we just haven't clicked.

I remember one instance when I went to her office to voice an annoyance. The office was as white as snow, spotless, very organized, very little clutter. As with almost every other office in the Rehabilitation Counseling Department, Mrs. Patterson's office had that one seat especially for the student. I eyed the brown chair with plastic armrests, a little wary for I didn't know if I should walk out of the office or proceed with my appointment.

I am always wary of the seat. I think the seat can be inviting if you are making a five-minute, hi and bye visit, but the same seat can be dangerous if you intend to inquire about a professor's reasoning for a poor grade or written criticism for more than ten minutes.

But, being the inexperienced, first year graduate student I am, I decided to question Mrs. Patterson. I never had a chance.

"I just think my grade is unfair," I said. "I made some small grammatical errors, but not enough to warrant a C+!"

"Are you telling me I'm mistaken?" Mrs. Patterson raised her eyebrow, her bright eyes boring into me. I wanted to say she was wrong, that everyone can be wrong at some point.

"I just think it is unfair, because overall, I wrote a good paper!" I became defensive, crossed my arms. "I need a better grade! Please!"

She leaned back in her chair, her hair bouncing as she tipped. "I warned you about the APA guidelines. Plagiarism is unacceptable." I didn't like that accusatory response. It made me feel small, as if I wasn't good enough.

"Chris," she said more sensitively. "Do you understand I gave you the grade because you need practice and can do better?"

I scowled at her, looked down at her immaculate desk. Inside, I knew I was going to blow up. I can't handle it when people don't acknowledge my hard work. "Screw the APA! Screw this! This whole conversation is pointless!"

Again in a softer tone, she said, "I'm sorry, Chris. But I'm not going to change my mind."

"Whatever."

That response got me nowhere. I learned shutting up was the best way to get by. My experience helped me empathize with Michael, as I now have to hold my tongue in my department. Since the meeting, though, Mrs. Patterson and I have learned to agree to disagree. I still hate the APA (American Psychological Association) writing format, and I still have my theory on the chair, but I have refined my communication style.

• • •

As MICHAEL and I walk away from the window and to the middle of the room to settle down, I conclude my concerns about communication and relationships, among other issues relating to my seizures, are almost nonexistent when my mind is elsewhere. Knowing this, I remember, at the start of the school year, Michael and I purchased a wide-screen television to clear our heads when necessary. We split the cost down the middle so it wouldn't empty our pockets, and we often watch it at night in the living room. We will tonight. I don't know about Michael, but I need to ease my feelings of tension.

Of course, studying is priority. Unfortunately. I can't empty my head until I have read, studied, or worked on papers for a while. Michael and I situate ourselves on the floor, and we begin deliberating over our assignments in silence. I always work hard, but I don't necessarily enjoy my efforts. I want to be carefree. Especially tonight, for my seizure has taken its toll.

I have seen Michael, on the other hand, works hard, and loves doing so. Even now. He will lie on his stomach and read and write with great interest, totally absorbed. I take the same position on the cheap carpeting and do the same thing, but whatever I read leaves my mind instantly. Clearly, Michael is a better student.

He has a pen behind his one ear always, and two highlighters behind his other. When he sees a valuable piece of information, he quotes a phrase for which he is known. "Hmmmm. Interesting." He then slides a highlighter from beneath his tuft of hair and marks the page. His Dad was a strong advocate of highlighting notable work when growing up, very strict about regiment. Often, his other highlighter will slide out of position, and fall to the ground. This annoys Michael, but I think it's funny and laugh anyway. He keeps on highlighting, and I can't help but admire his work ethic.

Tonight, a bag of Fritos separates us both, the smell of salty tortilla chips lingering in the air. We share the addictive treat; eat the whole bag usually. Despite the grease on my fingers, I type on my laptop. I skim my material for important quotes, and then reword them on my pc. I hate silence, and keep looking at my watch. When our hour is up, I think, *Thank God!*

Michael keeps reading but he speaks up. "You know, I haven't hosted my debate club in a while. I want to start up again." Michael is a very analytical person, and he likes to voice his opinions in a healthy setting. He listens to others share their stance, and then respectfully sorts through inconsistencies in their views, ultimately questioning its validity. His ability amazes me.

Perhaps the constant barrage of oppressive, religious reprimands at home impacted him so radically he thought it was better to question solid truths and embrace the unknown. He says no, but because I'm a counselor in training, I recognize the influence of atmosphere on a person transitioning into adulthood. In my opinion, this is basic stuff.

I ask him, "Wouldn't you rather join a club that considers the plausibility of multiple factors supporting a view? It would be much more positive that way." I have suggested this before, and he prefers to continue in his pessimism; just like some professors I know. Always in an acceptable environment, he emphasizes with a laugh. "It's fun!" he says. I smile, shaking my head. I'm not going to argue with him.

"Anyway . . . You ready for some Monday night football?" I ask. "Steelers are playing I think."

"Yeah. I think you're right." I quickly walk to my room, and return with my yellow, terrible towel.

GRAND MAL

"Go Pittsburgh." Michael says, putting his pen, highlighters, and books away, and pulling out the little black and gold foam football we throw around during the game.

Although he has retired, I cautiously yell, "Bettis all the way, baby!" Still recovering from my seizure, I don't feel like my normal self quite yet, and I don't want my excitement to induce any undue pain. Let me tell you, though, there is nothing like a good game on the tube to dull a headache, and clear my mind.

. . .

AFTER WATCHING television this night, I get in bed for some well-deserved relaxation. My mattress cradles me like a mother does her baby, and my head rests comfortably on a pillow of cotton clouds. I am a light sleeper and a heavy dreamer, and I hope to sleep well.

Before I fall asleep though, my mind starts to pace back and forth in a hall of memories. As it paces, it recalls times in my life, most of them upsetting. These times are upsetting because I didn't ask for them. I received unwanted attention for a condition I wish didn't exist. My condition, seizure activity as a result of Epilepsy, made me a focal point, a focal point that forced upon me more pressure to please, dependence, and initiated resentment towards others who expected gratitude for their so-called help.

Due to the disturbing nature of my condition, like many with disability-related impairments, I usually provoke confusion, apprehension, and ultimately fear in others. Except for Michael. Even in the most upsetting circumstances, at fourteen years old in seventh grade, he never lost his composure. He kindly pushed everyone else away, and laid my sweaty head in his lap.

I remember a girl named Mary Grace, a nice girl a year younger than us, who sat down next to Michael when he waited for me to come back to life. She always whispered, "It's all right Chris. Everything will be alright." If anyone else had said that, I would have been irritated beyond words, but she was angelic. She was all a boy could want, had blue eyes, long blond curly hair, a white dress, and a halo in my mind's eye. At the time, I didn't know her that well, but I knew she was a caring person who was not concerned with being popular, who had good grades, and who could become a good friend. "He will be alright," Michael always assured her, confidently rubbing his chin.

Looking back, despite having a faithful friend in Michael, and a supportive girl in Mary Grace, I worried constantly I would lose them and any future friends as a result of my seizures. I was different. I am still different. I had no way of telling whether the kids would avoid me because I could potentially interrupt their free time, and I'm not sure anyone would acknowledge this concern even today.

Persons, places, or events that make me worried, angry, or sad haunt me in various ways when I dream, and hypothetical possibilities emerge in rapid succession until I stop trying to sleep. A few of the biggest instigators of these dreams are the loss of friendship, rejection, and humiliation.

On these nights when my mind races, I do eventually tell myself, even though there haven't been many, I have had friends, and my mind slows to a jog.

GRAND MAL

• • •

A DAY AFTER my seizure, and an hour before lunch, I gather my materials and jog downtown to Starbucks for a flavored Chai tea. Inside, I hear Louie Armstrong on the radio, singing 'What a Wonderful World', one of my all-time favorites. Louie's raspy voice makes me feel light-hearted. I sit down and listen to the bluesy tune for a minute, then pull out my laptop. Usually, I play games on my computer, my preference either arcade or sports-related. I must be a funny sight, because I wince every time I lose or die. I do try to keep myself under control, but sometimes I could hop from my chair and scream out of frustration.

All about me, students are sitting at small tables, and have their hands wrapped around their mugs of coffee or tea. Some are studying. Some are talking with friends. Others are just thinking, casually passing away time. I am casually passing away time, too. Maybe not productively, however.

I am resorting to computer games instead of social and physical activities. For years now, I've settled for cartoons jumping and racing on a screen at my command as opposed to doing so myself, as opposed to participating in an activity with others. I could get too anxious or too overwhelmed, I've always thought, potentially causing a seizure.

I kind of want to take a risk though. Before my surgery, I did get involved in karate, and my seizure level decreased a great deal. I have frequently thought about the times I went to my karate class, and how good it made me feel. I want to have that feeling again.

And I can. Just down the street, on the way here, I saw a gym sign advertising a free karate lesson, and despite the safety precautions by which I should abide, I decide to check it out, to see if I can fight.

• • •

IT IS a fight getting through the door at Starbucks, but I make it outside, where students and faculty are chatting at round tables under green, Starbucks umbrellas. From there, I head to a busy place outdoors, art supplies in hand. I then sit under the summer sun with my pencil and drawing pad, to sketch people as they walk beneath the canopies of branches and leaves that hang from oaks all around.

Today, in particular, I sit on one of the benches that face the steps of Old Main, a beautiful building with a cobblestone exterior, several windows with cream-colored window frames, and a large steeple. Many group rallies are held here, so the surrounding courtyard is normally congested with people. For hours, I try to compose a portrait as I listen to the sounds of campus life, the university bell chime, the singing birds, the student conversations and laughter.

These days remind me how important drawing is to me. It is a form of therapy that alleviates my angst, and a release that allows me to express myself in a very personal way. When I was young, I enjoyed sharing my love for creativity with Michael, and he loved watching me.

We'd lay in my back yard, under a large tree with damaged bark. He would lay on his back, hands behind his head, resting in the soft soil, and look up at the oak's wooden fingers as I lay on my stomach, scanning my surroundings for an inspirational piece of nature to put on paper. Once I found what I wanted, I would run my idea by Michael, and he would either approve or make helpful suggestions.

As a beginning artist, I was a big fan of color experimentation. I still am. For a time, however, I worked with one main color. Michael was supportive of my artistic liberties, as well.

Back then, my seizures impacted my drawing style a great deal. During my teenage years, my seizures were accompanied by repeated nightmares of being shackled to a weight, falling in a never-ending whirlpool of clear blue water inside a gothic church. I would be submerged in liquid, drowning, gravity's death grip tugging from the depths. I would see stray Bibles and hymnals float on by me as I was sucked into a bottomless abyss of dark blues. With all the shades of blue in these dreams, I started using excess amounts of the color in my drawings. I remember Michael pushing his red hair out of his face, dirt caked on his forehead, and commenting on my change in style.

"You know, Chris, your drawings are much different than they used to be."

"It's just like in my seizures, Michael," I would say. "Really blue. Almost Van Gogh blue."

Michael didn't have an artistic eye, and still doesn't. However, when I was drawing in shades of blue that day, he sat up and said, "I'm gonna try to draw you a picture." I was thrilled he wanted to participate in my activity, so I gave him my pad to work on. Before I knew it, he had drawn an abstract looking girl with a halo above her head. He smiled. "I saw the way you were looking at Mary Grace in class today. Now you can look at her all day."

We laughed together a lot. Laughing with my only real friend, a rare but good memory. Outside Old Main again, I have an epiphany. I now know what I'll put on paper. I see a tall girl with curly blond ringlets in a white dress walk up the steps. The bell chimes as she reaches the last step and I press the tip of my pencil to the piece of paper.

• • •

WALKING ON Pollock Road, still thinking about the times I used blue in my art, I notice the blue tint of the sky isn't as bright as it was when I started drawing. White cumulus clouds have moved in, hiding much of the color. What a marvel, nature is.

Looking at the clouds consume the sky, slowly moving ahead, something else occurs to me. I haven't seen my doctor forever. Huh. Well how does my mind go from blue pastel work to nature to my doctor, you ask? The pills I take are blue. It's almost too ironic.

I'm on three medications, actually, but I'm not certain how effective the blue pill, Depakote ER, is. I would like to speak with my neurologist about other options. While I do not entirely trust him, I make a mental note to give the doctor a call when I get home.

First though, under the cover of clouds, I am going to go to the HUB.

• • •

ON A regular basis, I go to the HUB Robeson building, the center of activity, where all the undergraduates usually mingle. All the restaurants on the ground floor, Italian, Chinese, and fast food, are available to the students for most of the day. I prefer the fast food.

It is important for me to be around the hustle and bustle, the fast paced routine of academic life. Otherwise, I waste time in my room, bored to tears because I don't know what to do with myself. Despite the constant flow of kids who meander haphazardly, and the loiterers in the lobby, I find the HUB the most relaxing place on campus.

It is a three-tiered structure. I usually sit in the lounge area on the first floor, below the second and third floor offices. Several green chairs are set sporadically so students and teachers who are tired can rest, eat, watch news on the big screen television, or use the hot spots to work on their laptops, allowing them to finish up assignments. I bring my laptop with me, and cross my fingers in hopes of a free electric socket for my charger.

It's not surprising I have to write a lot of papers. After all, I am in graduate school. It is nice to have a place like the HUB to type up grants and summaries of specific research styles.

When I'm not doing this, however, I find a chair hidden behind one of the artificial planters, and I close my eyes and reflect.

I think about the bumpy roller coaster I rode at age nine, the wind rustling my hair with its gusty hands, the bumps, twists, and turns on the tracks that caused the return of my seizures. After five years of normalcy, of perfect physical health, I convulsed violently after the ride. My family and I were devastated.

We had planned to spend a relaxing day at an amusement park, which we did; we watched caricature artists make funny pictures of

people, we ate hotdogs and various sweets provided by street vendors, and we played games, my favorite being ski ball because the
clown laughed at me when I missed the holes. We never thought,
though, a wooden construct meant to entertain would bring our fun
to a halt, and cause me any harm. This occurrence preceded years
of hospital visits.

The lounge area is normally relaxing, but today it is getting
claustrophobic. To my left, an older gentlemen has opened the
school newspaper, *The Daily Collegian*, to glance at the weekly edi-
torials, a girl to my right is curled up in a fetal position sleeping, and
right in front of me, a young man is playing with a new iPod, his
headphones blaring. I really need to go. There is a Barnes & Noble
bookstore in the basement of the HUB, thank God. So I shut down
my laptop, and walk towards the stairs that lead there. It is busy in
the basement too, I know, but there are books. My favorite.

• • •

BEFORE I even get to the stairs, though, I see some of Michael's
colleagues. I can tell they are checking out a girl, because they are
whistling, then nudging each other in the ribs, and then laughing
with one another, still stealing glances at her as she walks ahead of them.

I think, *No wonder women think men are pigs. But, you know, who can
blame us? There are so many beauties at this university!* I steal a few glances
myself, but am interrupted when the guys approach me, yelling out,
"Hey! Chris!"

I say, "Hey guys. What's goin' on?"

John, Michael's good friend, says, "So Chris, we were gonna go to the Deli this weekend. You open to coming? Michael said he was." He shifts on his feet, as antsy as a toddler. I've heard he always has to move about. And I think I recall Michael telling me he was like a real Forrest Gump growing up, always running from bullies, which makes sense.

If I remember correctly, John's mother was a teacher, and when any of his peers earned a bad grade, a day in detention, or a visit to the principal's office, he took the brunt. He was in a rough spot, resents his mother for it, I think, and it is, unfortunately, very apparent today. His nerves are fried.

"That would be great." I smile, thinking, *Hmmm. Wow. Someone actually wants me to be a part of something.*

John taps his feet on the floor, obviously eager to reply. "We'll have to give Michael a hard time about the girl he's been talking to."

"He's interested in this girl?" I question, shocked.

"Oh yeah." He laughs, instigating laughs from Alex, one of the other guys making a scene.

Alex is an overweight fellow with beady eyes, a stubby nose, and rosy cheeks. His receding hairline reveals numerous creases in his forehead. When picking on others, he bursts with hilarity, and his creases fissure like uneven ground during an earthquake. His forehead moves back and forth when he asks, "You didn't know?"

I don't like the tone in Alex's voice and I'm about to say something sarcastic about his weight, but I hold my tongue. Michael also told me not to be offended by Alex's behavior. I guess, growing up, he didn't know his parents, jumped from foster home to foster home, his only relatives his grandparents, both of whom made fun of him. Unfortunately, while Alex resented his grandparents, he learned from them the art of verbal abuse, and uses it to make himself feel better. Good old human nature for you.

I find it so interesting how people adjust behaviors to adversities in life, and continue to maintain the same behaviors after the hardships have ended. Whereas John ran away from his problems and developed nervous habits, Alex confronted his adversaries by belittling them.

I don't respond to Alex's question but I bet there are a few creases on my forehead. I turn to leave. Close by, at the information desk, a ticket sales person from the Bryce Jordan Center is distributing tickets to as many students as possible, to clear the long line preventing me from moving. Perhaps *Hairspray*, the Broadway musical, has come to town. Musicals seem to be popular here at Penn State.

As I continue to make my way downstairs, I am still awestruck by the fact I didn't know about Michael's love life. It is big news to me.

• • •

Inside BARNES & Noble, I pass the girl at the cash register, the selection of school materials, the frame display, the assortment of officially licensed hats, sweatshirts, sweatpants, and more, and go to the shelf holding all the new nonfiction novels.

Ironically, I find a black book about a person with a disability, an inspirational sort. The inside of the cover gives a brief synopsis of a blind man who climbs a mountain, his difficulties and successes, a real dynamic tale.

I stand here quietly in my Penn State paraphernalia, trying to avoid nearby shoppers, and flip through the beginning pages, skimming over the preface and reading the prologue. It is a story that captures my attention, and I want to buy it. No money, unfortunately. It inspires me, though, to tell my story. I sure haven't climbed a mountain, but I have lived through a big setback.

The seizures led to a one-month stay in the neurology department at John Hopkins hospital. I remember the smell of disinfectant, of alcohol, and bad hospital food. I remember smelling of sweat because I didn't bathe daily, and of iodine at times.

I recall the small size of the hospital room, how most of my family and visitors had to stand when they came to see me. Yes, there were chairs, but very few, forcing visitors to take turns if they wanted to sit. There was a small TV bolted to one yellow, concrete wall for their entertainment, but with all the nurses checking on me, no one could really enjoy a movie or show. There was a window that made the room feel a little more open.

I remember lying in the motorized hospital bed, cold, bare, and vulnerable, my skin as white as the anesthesiologist's latex gloves. In my little hospital dress, making sure the IV in my arm didn't get in the way, I tried to conceal myself under the green blankets.

In my most vulnerable state, I met my friend Michael. He was in the room across the hall from me, and he was almost ready to leave the hospital for good, only a week to go. His surgery was successful. No more medicines needed, no more special diets, no more seizures.

Sometimes when Michael and I sit in the living room of our apartment now, I ask him why he thinks his surgery was successful, and why mine was not. We haven't yet come to a reasonable conclusion.

We both have the same scars marking our heads, and we both share traumatic memories, but his life improved, and mine took a turn for the worse. In the end, we agree my circumstances could be the basis for the universal question of why bad things happen to good people.

I recollect the first day I was permitted to leave the hospital room, in a wheelchair pushed by one of my parents or grandparents, all of whom took turns staying with me. I saw Michael in the corridor with his Mom, who happened to be carrying a King James Version Bible. One of the accompanying nurses waved Michael in my direction and introduced him to me shortly after.

"I hope your surgery helps you Chris," I remember Michael saying after we hung out for a week, becoming immediate friends. "I really do."

With no fear, or absolute naivety, I said, "I hope so, too."

"When you get out, maybe we can play." That thought made me happy. And that's how our bond originated. We traded addresses and promised to stay in touch. He left shortly after, and I wrote him daily until medical procedures occupied most of my time.

In the next couple of weeks, I went through several painful tests, medicinal experiments, and long meetings with the surgeons. I was excited at times. I was unsure at times. But mostly, I was miserable.

Before I went into the surgery room very early in the morning on "the big day", my head was shaven clean but free of any hurt.

When I was rolling down the hall, I said to my parents, "God will be with me." And He was and is. But He allowed a great deal of suffering. When I came out of surgery twelve hours later, my head was wrapped in a turban, as if I had been born in the Middle East. The wrapping held my skull together, knotted so tight the firm cloth hammered nails of pain above and behind my tender ears.

I was warned there was a possibility I might die under the knife. My parents and I took the risk, signing the contract. Obviously, I am still here. I fought the fight, reading, writing, and drawing to take my mind off of my hospital stay.

I read a book then, and I am reading a book now. The blind mountain climber survived, and so have I.

• • •

WHEN I arrive at the Deli, I don't have the book about the mountain climber on me, but I see a menu I can peruse. Michael is on his way. John, Alex, and some other guys I don't know are already here. They are sitting at a booth nearby, so I bypass the customers in line, grab the menu, and look at it as I head to where they are. I am eager to learn more of the girl Michael is talking to, and curious to see how Michael will respond to the jabs his colleagues will most likely inflict, all in good fun of course.

To be honest, I'm just glad I'm at this restaurant. In my opinion, it is the best culinary establishment in State College. The Deli is a part bar, part formal restaurant. It satisfies both the frequent student customers, and the occasional, visiting parents. The food is just great, and the flavored, Hawaiian tea is unlike any you will find in town.

I am hungry, so I say hello to everyone, sit down, call over the waitress, and order the Deli's classic potato soup. The guys are laughing, nudging each other, and staring at a girl again, another waitress, as she walks into the kitchen. She has a smirk on her face, too.

John says, "She's a looker, huh Chris?" I smile, sort of embarrassed.

"Yeah." I say softly, trying not to let her hear. "She's pretty." They all chuckle at my response. Especially Alex. He adds, "True. True," a comment I'd later learn he adds to every response he gives.

"Glad you came," John says. "Wanted you to be here to celebrate Michael's find." John is a small guy, very comparable to myself, actually. But a similar stature is all we have in common. Whereas I have a goatee and a thick head of dark brown hair, John's face is bare, and his head is totally bald.

"Me too." I say. "It's always fun to be with friends." Inside, I am still wondering why Michael hasn't told me. I then look around, and I reconsider whether this place should be classified as formal, or more pop-culture. It can be both, really. The tables have candles in the center, and the napkins are shaped like fans, but on the walls, a big golden bull head is mounted, a picture of Betty Boop covers a large space, and objects like sleds, coke bottles, and barber shop signs hang, almost placing me back in the Norman Rockwell era. I really wouldn't look all that out of place here if I read the old *Saturday Evening Post.*

Michael arrives when my potato soup comes out. I couldn't have planned it better myself. He grabs a chair from another table, and sits at the head of the four-top. "Hmmm. Very interesting crew, here."

"True. True," Alex says, his fat thumbs pointing upwards. "How's the new love of your life, Mikey?"

"She's fine," Michael says. "It's nothing serious, yet."

"Yet?" John replies, laughing and stomping his feet on the ground. "Yet? Did you hear that guys? There's a yet!" They all give each other high fives. I offer a high five, even though I'm not excited like the rest of them.

Michael blushes, goes red in the face. "Honestly. Just hanging out with her for now."

"Hanging out with her where?" John asks, insinuating something I don't even want to think of.

"Yeah! Where?" the rest of them chime in. The jabbing continues, and Michael gets redder and redder. I enjoy myself, but then I remember I have other things to accomplish. So, I finish my soup, and get up.

"Gotta go, guys. Had fun." I say, giving handshakes to them all. I have a hard time fitting my hand around Alex's stubby fingers. Poor kid. "I've got a paper due in my psychosocial class tomorrow."

• • •

AFTER I finish my paper, sitting on an uncomfortable, wooden chair before my desktop computer, I pick up my phone from its cradle, my fingers sore from typing, and punch in the number to my doctor's office. I know he has gone home for the day, and probably is not on call, but I intend to leave a message.

Outside my nearby window, I see it is starting to rain. The white sidewalk leading to the front entrance of my apartment gradually turns a shade of gray as the once dry concrete pads soak up the water droplets. The parking lot is filling up too, each pothole in the pavement overflowing. It is a good night to be inside.

I listen to the phone ring until an answering machine picks up. It takes a while, but I eventually hear the recorded voice of my doctor's secretary ask me to be specific with my information. I begin speaking after the beep.

"Hello, this is Chris. Just wanted to talk to the doctor about my seizures, and to see if he will help me in adjusting my dosage, or changing it all together. Thanks." I relay my phone number and time I should be in.

The wind rattles the walls of my room, and the rain picks up speed. It is so relaxing.

• • •

ON THE days I have my psychosocial class, I have to take the red and white CATA bus from my apartment to the campus. The ride is short, maybe five minutes. However, at times, depending how full the bus is, it feels longer. The transportation service is great, but I don't think CATA considers the comfort of their customers.

On a more positive note, while many of the drivers lack enthusiasm, they are timely. I punctually arrive at the first on-campus stop, at the Patee-Paterno library. The library towers over me. Four beige light posts make the front doors highly visible, and a pine green, life-size abstract gives an ultra-modern effect. The lilacs in the nearby stone planters emit a fresh scent. I marvel at Joe Paterno's generosity, for donating so much money to improve the overall quality of the structure.

I observe the students as they stand under the concrete columns that support the square overhang. They read or smoke when they aren't studying inside, and hide from the rain if they are waiting on a ride. I then walk to the Counselor Education building. I travel on foot about five minutes, pass the Chambers building, the brick College of Education sign wrapped in mulch and flowers, and then follow the sidewalk to the CEDAR building entrance. As I make this daily walk I think about my irritating transportation predicament. I've always had the predicament.

Because of my seizure disorder, I have never had the opportunity to drive. I never experienced the excitement of driving a car on my sixteenth birthday. I was so envious of Michael because he was able to do what I couldn't, own a car. To have to ask others to take me places was and continues to be awful, dark thoughts of this fact claw at my psyche. As you might have noticed, I am already a passive person, an introvert who thinks about things that trouble me. An inability to take myself to certain places by myself is a constant reminder of what able-bodied people can do on a regular basis, and of what I cannot. When I have to depend on another person's wheels, I feel like a burden.

In middle school, if friends or family members promised to take me places, and they changed their minds, or circumstances arose that disrupted the plans, I would be ticked. My anger would then turn to sadness. *Why does this always happen to me?* I would think. I also feared upsetting my family members and friends because I didn't know how my responses would affect my daily plans. My plans could be ruined by a look, a facial expression, a reluctant word. It is still a worry.

No time to worry now though. It is time to work. Once inside the CEDAR building, I walk up three flights of stairs to the top floor, and delve into a long white corridor where offices with closed wooden doors on either side conceal the professors within. My class is in a conference room at the end of the hall, just beyond the offices. I take in a deep breath and blow out, preparing myself for a three-hour discussion on disability.

• • •

I HAVE TO admit talking about disability culture in general feels strange to me since I do have a condition that places me within this particular culture. Unlike some with my disorder, I don't like acknowledging the accompanying stigma, much less accepting it for what it is. Why make an issue out of it?

"Disability culture is such an important issue in our field." My professor, Miss Love, reminds me. "After all, we as counselors have to understand psychosocial aspects, how our client will respond to us, and what makes them respond the way they do."

I look around the conference room. It is a small room, all white except for a few flyers taped to the wall advertising Chi Sigma Iota (honor society) events. In the center, my colleagues and I sit around a glossy, mahogany table with our text and notebooks in front of us. There are eleven of us, all of whom are unique and different, sarcastic and fun, but also analytical and critical thinkers.

In hopes of not being called on again, I say, "I agree." And I leave it at that.

Talking for three hours can be tedious. Normally, I participate so I learn more, keeping in mind it will pass the time more quickly as well, but this topic is not one of my favorites, so I drift off.

I think about what really contributed to my perceived place in society. Yes, I had seizures before adolescence, but my hospital visits and eventual brain surgery really sealed the deal. The types of seizures and new intensity of the brain activity after surgery changed my life. Looking back, it was about power. I think it's safe to say power is involved in every person's place in society, but when it comes to my disability, my seizures, and the doctors and surgeons involved, I was like a leaf thrown about in the wind, an experiment in a test tube passed from hospital to hospital. To think now that men in white coats played God, that they sat behind closed doors and discussed the implications of mistakes in surgery, and their own improved reputations if I was a success story is disturbing. It unnerves me sixteen years later.

Teresa, an intelligent girl and a regular participant with experience in social work says, "In my view, if you analyze culture too much, you will stereotype persons with disabilities. Possibly distort their identities. Limit their successes, too." Amen.

My black, leather bag rests at my feet under the table. It is almost break time, and I plan to get a snack and a soda. I pull out some money from my wallet and hold it in my hands. On one of the flyers, I see a party will be held soon. At the bottom of the flyer, there is a black and white photo of a table with a platter of food spread before several members of the honor society. My stomach growls, a hungry feline in my body.

Before the discussion moves forward, I say, "All I know is that I don't want my minority status to determine who I am." My professor nods.

I then hear Miss Love say, "Let's take our break. Twenty minutes. Be back here."

• • •

ON OCCASION, popular bands will come to town, and if I have the money, I will rush to buy the tickets, relishing the thought of having the ridged pieces of paper between my fingers. The same tickets that excite me, though, also make me nervous at times. I guess it's the fear of losing the tickets, and the responsibility to keep an eye on them so I can take a break from the heavy workload that can be so burdensome.

I think about this when, after my psychosocial class, one of the girls says to the entire group, "We should all go to a concert sometime." The idea doesn't go over real well. I am disappointed, but, later, when I am over at the Weston Community Center picking up my mail, I notice a flyer with my favorite band on the front, the date they are coming, and the cost of the show. Inside, I am thinking, *Yes! Sweet!*

The tickets usually have a sale date, notifying me of the day I need to pick them up. I hate to admit it, but I know from experience that, if you aren't one of the first to get to the ticket office, you don't get the good seats. Fortunately for me, the sale date this year falls on a free day, a day of no classes. So I plan to walk to the ticket office.

The Performing Arts building is all the way across campus, a long way for me to walk. I need some personal time, though. I know it. And if I don't allow myself a relaxing evening every once in a while, I might burn out. Whatever it takes is worth it.

Last year, the line was incredibly long, a slithering snake with a winding tail. It is just as long this year, if not longer, and I stand here for about two hours, moving forward as slow as a bored slug. About halfway to the ticket booth, the line comes to a halt, one of many halts, and I shuffle on my feet like John, looking at a framed board of signatures from all the famous bands that have come to town. I marvel at all the musicians' handwriting until it is my turn at the ticket booth.

• • •

NEARING THE door of my apartment, tickets in my pocket, I hear laughter. Michael's laughter. And a girl's laughter. It is surprising to hear a female voice in our pad, and my curiosity peaks. I put my hand on the knob to open the door, but it won't open. It is locked. Unusual. I consider knocking, but decide not to. Pulling out my key, and inserting it into the keyhole, I unlock the door, allowing me to enter.

I peek my head inside. "Yo!"

"Oh hey, Chris," Michael says. "How's it goin'?"

"Good." I reply. "Who's our visitor here?"

The girl is smiling broadly, hiding behind Michael. "This is Linda."

Linda is a petite girl, has long auburn hair, deep brown eyes, and a cute, crooked grin. She has stylish cat glasses balanced on a cute little nose, and a subtle hint of red lipstick on her lips. *Michael has good taste*, I think. "Hi," she says.

"Hi. Nice to meet you." I smile. When she turns away, I mouth to Michael, 'Dang! She's hot!'

I then turn, go into my room. Talk and laughter seeps under the crack in my door like an infectious gas. This continues for a couple of hours, and then all is still. When she leaves, I go out into the kitchen where Michael is cooking an Indian dish, the smell burning my nostrils. "That smells so bad, man," I say.

"But it tastes awesome. An interesting flavor," he counters. It gets quiet a minute, but, seconds later, Michael breaks the silence. "By the way, Linda told me to tell you again it was nice meeting you."

"Okay," I say. "Well thanks, I guess." I walk over to the table, and push all the chairs in. "Hey. I'm curious. Where did you meet her?"

"Met her at a restaurant. I complimented on her hair, some of her jewelry. The next thing I know, she is on break, we are talking. She tells me she is a philosophy major. I tell her I love that area of study, and we talk forever about it. We've been hanging out since." He rubs his goatee, scratches his thick unibrow. "I think we are going to go to the Dave Matthews Band concert."

"Me too. I just got back from the ticket office. Maybe you can give me a lift."

"I don't know, man. You don't think you'll have a seizure do you?" he asks. "I don't want Linda to see you have one. It might scare her away."

"You know as well as I do that I don't know when they are gonna happen. What if I do have one?" I question. "Will you avoid me to spare your girlfriend?"

He is silent, and his lack of a response makes me question our friendship.

• • •

THAT QUESTION and lack of a response upsets me. And to ease my angry feelings, I leave Michael be for a little while. During this time, though, I repeatedly tell myself I am being unreasonable, and I eventually ask him if he will accompany me to a couple places. I want him to hang with me at the Kern Graduate Building for a time, and then go down town to the gym where the karate classes are being offered. He agrees to come with me.

We opt to walk over to campus, so we are presently approaching the large walkway, a bridge above the main thoroughfare if you will, that allows us to pass over North Atherton Street. As we cross the bridge, we look at the classrooms behind glass on either side. There is a deli on the left side with a large area for everyone to sit. The Dell computer store and an art exhibit are a few steps away. On the right side, there is another lounge, and just beyond it are a Xerox copy store and the Apple computer store. It is an amazing construct. We reach the end of the bridge a minute later. We are both winded.

"Tired?" I ask Michael.

He heaves. And then he fibs. "Not a chance!"

• • •

FROM THERE we walk up Burrowes Road, a shady street lined with colonial-style fraternity and sorority houses, pass a CATA bus, the White Loop, and Waring Commons. The Kern building is around the corner from the Commons and catty corner to the Recreation Building. Inside Kern, it is packed. The vestibule opens up into a large space where several round and square tables are separated by only a foot or so. Students and faculty rush to grab the empty tables nearest to them. Long flags with the logos of all the teams we play in the Big Ten conference hang from the ceiling, and I count them, focusing on the represented teams we still haven't played this season.

Michael tugs at my arm. "There's a free table over there! Hurry or we'll lose it!"

I say, "Awesome. Perfect timing." We jog over to a table high off the ground with a set of high stools, and place our bags and coats there to save our spot.

Once he has grabbed a bagel and a caramel latte, and I have grabbed a donut and Chai tea, we awkwardly settle on our stools. I am about to apologize for getting annoyed, when he silences me. "Don't worry about it," he says. "I was the ass."

"I was just being immature." There is a curved, Indian-like pattern on the table, and I stare at it, moving my finger in a circular motion over the glazed outline.

Michael says, "It's just that she's talking to me about heavy stuff. Like long term stuff for us. Her future with me." He looks around us, trying to keep his voice low.

"Already?" I say, looking up from the table, stopping my finger motions. "I just heard you were talking to her."

"We've been talking a long time. I just decided not to tell you. Sorry." He waves his hand in the air to emphasize what he is saying. In doing so, I see a small cross tattoo under his wrist that has a red banner with the word LOVE over it. He must have had it done recently, within the past month. I think, *Man oh man, will his parents tell him he's going to hell!* But I don't say anything, for the tattoo convinces me my friend is telling the truth.

To some extent, I appreciate his honesty, so I reply, "No. It's all right. I understand."

$$\bullet \ \ \bullet \ \ \bullet$$

I DO UNDERSTAND. I probably would do the same if my friend would be upset by the news. So I don't make an issue of it again. *Enough of this serious talk*, I think. *Let's have fun!* Judging from the perplexed yet hopeful expression on his face, I sense Michael agrees with me. We talk about some lighter topics while finishing up our sweets, and then leave the Kern building.

Almost forty-five minutes later, we enter the side door to the gym offering karate lessons. Our earlier talk no longer an issue. We find the office immediately. It is small, but acceptable, considering the gym isn't all that large either. On the main wall, two swords are mounted on either side of a glass encasement. The encasement glistens, protecting several large trophies. Behind a nicked table, a muscular guy with a long braided ponytail reclines in a leather chair, manning a nearby phone, and, I assume, working on finances. He asks how he can help us.

I smile and put out my hand for a shake. "I am interested in the martial arts class you are offering." He shakes my hand, almost breaks it actually (unlike Alex's shake, let me tell you!), pulls out a pamphlet, and points out with his free hand the good deals.

"Most likely I'll do the group class, but I'd like to take the free lesson first."

"Good. Good. Wise choice," he says in an authoritative, Mr. Miyagi way. Looking down at my throbbing open hand, he places the pamphlet in my palm, and then pulls at his ponytail, wrapping it up into a bun. "And what about your friend here?"

I turn to Michael. "A free lesson man. You can't beat it."

"Yeah. I guess you're right." We both make arrangements and head out with another thing to look forward to.

• • •

IN MID-JULY, the State College Arts Fest brings a lot of people to the Happy Valley. I have not experienced all the events and spectacles that make this annual festival so notorious. So, I am walking down College Avenue, passing several old houses hidden by shadows, observing students on the porches lounge, drink, and smoke. Typical activities at a party school.

About twenty houses later, I reach a mid-section where North Atherton Street and College Avenue intersect. I cross it, walk straight ahead into the thick of things, the restaurants and shops. Normally, the students parade into stores like Abercrombie & Fitch, Eddie Bauer, McClannahan's, and Webster's bookstore. During Arts Fest week, though, with all the tents placed everywhere, and a wide array of artistic merchandise available, pottery, paintings, and jewelry, the students migrate instead to these attractions.

When I reach Allen Street, I pass the Grille, an old restaurant with decent food, looking for a nearby bench. The street is blocked off, and a stage has been erected in the middle of the road. Several people are already sitting on benches, tapping their feet as one of the local, bluegrass cover bands plays an interesting version of an Elvis hit. I enjoy the concert, sitting in a good spot that permits me to see the entire concert unobstructed. It is something different.

I am hot, real sweaty, but I want to see everything down town. When the concert ends, I decide to walk around a little more. I see students on the roofs of their Allen Street apartments observing the masses as they maneuver their way along the sidewalks. I hear children squealing, and I smell chlorinated water. I am curious, and before long, I see a platform with moving buckets of water overhead. The children don't know which bucket will tip first, so they run as fast as they can in circles to avoid the liquid content in the rotating containers. I smile to myself, enjoying the carefree atmosphere.

I near a mist machine, walk through it to cool off, and observe several food stands, lemonade stands, and smoothie stands, a sweet lover's paradise. A jazz record plays over the speakers, sounding until the next musician is ready to perform. I get a milkshake at a nearby ice cream shop, and decide to head home. I am glad I went, and will return to the Arts Fest later this weekend.

• • •

ONLY UNTIL I walk out of the elevator just outside my apartment door do I forget Michael's debate team will be having a group session. Why they chose to do this over hanging with the masses at Arts Fest is beyond me, but I guess each person places value on something different. *What a shame*, I think.

If I remember correctly, the topic at hand is Plato and the allegory of the man who twice enters the cave with all the slaves.

I decide I'll sit with them. I have nothing else to do, and I might as well observe why Michael hosts this particular activity. You know, I have already stated why I believe he joined this group. His family life. To spite his parents. What I am still not convinced about is whether he enjoys questioning truth. He says so, but I find it hard to believe someone who once lived by absolutes, no matter how stringent, can, later in life, fully be content as a relativist.

By now, Michael, John, and Alex have moved our kitchen table out into the hall, and have set up the couches so they can face one another. The couches are bland and hard, a dull shade of grey with pillows that feel like wood. But it'll have to do. And the table! It is bent. A tree would be embarrassed! Nevertheless, they are all settled and ready to begin.

"So," Linda says, her cat glasses at the tip of her nose. "Where did we leave off?"

Michael says, "At the most interesting part! The cave and the shadows." His one thick eyebrow goes up like a puppy's ear when waiting on a treat. He then feels the highlighter behind his ear, his father's regimented training so obvious.

Linda eloquently says, "Yes. When these chained people are in the dark and can only see their shadows. For them, it is the only reality that exists."

"Hmmmm. Yet there are more than the shadows." Alex retorts antagonistically, wagging his pudgy finger in the air, his forehead extremely creased. "There is a wall, a fire, and wanderers with jars in hand. They don't help them, but they are also in the cave. Ha! So, there you go! Another reality!"

"So, what is real?" asks John, a bit edgy in his seat. "What is the truth?"

"That is the question John. That is why we are here!" says Michael, who I notice is making sure his watch covers the tattoo.

And so they all begin pondering these questions. They banter some, and I hear Alex say, "True" several more times. I get aggravated not only by his mantra, but also at the pointless nature of debating. What purpose does it serve?

I wonder about this for a reason. From experience, I know the die-hard analyst, whether it is a member of the press or an educated average Joe, likes to take a truth, and tear it apart so there is no reliable explanation for the subject in question. And what is interesting to me, and I have seen it repeatedly, on TV and here at school, is the fact that, in the end, some of the analysts don't really know what they believe, if in fact they ever did. And that, in my opinion, is reality.

When the debaters are done talking about the allegory, they relate the same principles to their own lives.

Alex says, "My definition of a good Parent is obviously different than my own Parents' definition. And my idea of verbal abuse is different than the ideas of my Grandparents."

"Along the same lines, Alex," John replies, shaking his head in agreement. "My Parents and I believe my peers at school abused me to get back at my Mother, but my bullies might have been doing it because they were cruel by nature. Who knows?"

Linda says, "Well. Plato's allegory gives us plenty to think about. That's for sure."

I agree. And from what I gather, the man in the allegory comes out of the cave more confused about reality than when he went inside, the sun beating down on him as he tries to reach enlightenment and find the truth.

• • •

THE SUN beats down on me, the light reflecting off my glasses like a mirror shimmering against a vase. I squint, cup my hands around my eyes to see through the strobes, and head for the shadows to ward off the heat. The air is still, no breeze at all, the Happy Valley as arid as a desert. It has been dry for a while, and a change in the weather is inevitable. I see cumulus clouds in the distance. *It's going to storm*, I think. *It's just a matter of time.*

On Allen Street again, I see the storeowners and employees are taking advantage of all the tourists visiting State College for the Arts Fest. They have set up outdoor clothing racks and boxes full of over-stocked hats, shorts, shirts, sweatshirts, sweatpants, and even jackets. Prices range from five dollars to seventy-five dollars. Not bad, I guess. As I look through the selection, though, I can't help but wonder whether the retailers jacked up the initial costs to make all of these items look like a steal. I guess they would be stupid not to.

So I won't spend money carelessly, I walk towards campus to see the talented artists from around the country manning more tents. Artists who sell some products at unimaginable prices. There are so many items and trinkets here at Arts Fest it could take multiple visits to see everything. I do manage to see a lot, however.

• • •

ONCE I'VE finished looking around the remaining tents on campus, I am inspired to draw. I have seen abstract lithographs, beautiful photography, impressionistic landscape paintings, and realistic portrait drawings. While I am eager to get my creative juices flowing, I wait, and return to Webster's bookstore. I spend hours here, no matter the time, weather, or season.

I have my own favorite section of the bookstore, a remote area towards the back in a cubicle-shaped box of bookshelves. I sit on a small bench, and swivel my body around to survey the used, but average, selection of novels. I soak up the smell of the novels, the pungent, sour odor of mildewed paper. A nasty smell to some, but a familiar and appreciated scent for me.

I also smell hot chocolate, cappuccino, and fruit. The smell is coming from the front of the building. "Mmmmmmmmm," I mutter to myself. *Man, I could go for a smoothie.* I haven't yet had one today, so I decide to get the treat. Besides, I have to go up front anyway, to talk to Sam, a mentor of mine.

On my way to the front of the store, I look at a variety of average pictures on the walls by some local artist I've never heard of. A different series of pictures is placed on the same walls weekly, and I wonder whether Sam would allow me to showcase my own artwork at some point. Not to be cocky, but I think I am a lot better than this guy.

Anyway, in the front of the store, Sam stands behind a coffee bar, a small café. He has thick glasses, a goatee, and long dreads that drape over his tie-dye shirt. He is sort of eccentric, loud, and loose with his tongue. I sometimes think he spikes his coffee and over-drinks, but he has always been nice to me, a good conversationalist who offers good advice.

I usually come here to write my master's paper on my laptop, to escape the miserable weather and relax, but, today, I have come to hear Sam's take on Michael's comment about my seizing in front of his girlfriend. I swivel in my little corner for about an hour, but I eventually walk to the front of the store and find a table to sit at, only a short distance away from the coffee bar.

No one is giving Sam business today, so I purchase the smoothie, a strawberry ice cream drink. Sam brings the smoothie over to me in his bare feet, limping. He was injured in Vietnam, was shot in the knee. His shoulders sag, his weariness obvious. He says, "What's happenin' young chap?"

"Nothing much. Just enjoying the Arts Fest."

"I bought a new bike, ya know." I shake my head in awe. This man is something. He has a big Cadillac at home, but he chooses to cycle to work everyday. In sandals! "I customized it," he goes on. "Looks like a Harley now." He chuckles as he pulls a chair out to sit with me. He props his leg up on a nearby table.

A rich man, Sam sees no reason to make a show of it. He inherited his riches, and he could easily act aloof, as if he is above us all. But he isn't. His humility is refreshing to those who know him. It is refreshing to me. Yet because he doesn't display his worth, he lost his wife, who evidently married him for his money.

To make his life even emptier, his wife took Sam's kid away. She filed for custody, after he returned from war, and won. He never saw him again, despite his efforts to get visitation. All Sam has left are memories from when his son was young. He has repeatedly told me he wished he had adopted after the divorce.

"A Harley?" I say. "Good for you. Your other bike was looking pretty pitiful." He emphatically nods. Looking down, I glance at his deformed leg, but turn away so I don't appear to be staring. I add, "Now all you need are some shoes."

"No way, lad. Shoes are for sissies." I look at his leg again. Sam once told me his wife had changed when he came home "a cripple". He believes she expected him to die and resented she couldn't live as a wealthy widow. This makes me sad for him.

"Tell me, Sam," I say. "Has anyone ever insinuated he or she wouldn't hang with you because of your injury?"

"One of the guys I shot in Vietnam!" He guffaws.

"No. Seriously."

"I guess. My ex-wife actually," he says. "I never really acknowledge rude people, though."

"My best friend is falling for a girl, and I think he wants me to stay away because of my seizures." I think, *Well he denied it, but still.*

Sam looks at an antique painting that hangs on the wall behind me. "Don't let it get you down, chap. You are too strong for that."

"But he's my best friend . . ." I take a deep breath, inhale deeply, and a waft of mildew and coffee envelopes me.

"Friends will come and go," he says. "As the saying goes, seasons change."

• • •

PART TWO:

FALL SEMESTER SEASONS CHANGE

SAM WAS right about the changing seasons, for summer has ended and fall is beckoning. The sun has stopped shining on a frequent basis and the wind calls out as rain falls, thunder rolls, and lightning cracks. The temperature is dropping. The students, myself included, no longer wear short-sleeved shirts. I have pulled out my black pea coat.

People aren't smiling as they do in the summer, the weather pretty depressing. I see many people running to their cars under umbrellas, squinting, and I am now one of those students keeping dry under the Patee-Paterno Library overhang, waiting for the CATA bus to arrive.

The green leaves on the trees have turned shades of gold, orange, and red. The leaves that have fallen from the oak canopies suffocate the earth's surface, preventing the grass to breathe, yellowing the reeds as they wither.

I hate getting out of bed some mornings.

One thing, however, that lifts my spirits is the opening of football season, watching the improved players I saw at the Blue and White game, at the pep rallies at the Recreation Building and Beaver Stadium. One day, sometime in June, when it was still summer, I also bought season tickets to watch the Nittany Lion football team play. Considering season tickets sell so quickly, I was fortunate.

When we play our most rivaled nemesis, the Ohio State Buckeyes, hordes of people, small children, adolescents, college students, parents, and grandparents, flood the sidewalks. Some of them walk down Curtin, Bigler, and Pollock Roads at a vigorous pace, in attempts to be the first to arrive at the front gates of Beaver Stadium.

There are always people scalping tickets outside the front gates, most of whom will hold the tickets up in the air waving them back and forth, calling out, "Selling tickets here!" Some will negotiate the sale price; some won't budge. It enlivens the atmosphere.

Every couple of feet, there are Penn State Bookstore stands filled with shirts, hats, cups, cheering items, and school programs. The sales representatives are running around disheveled, trying to keep up, gathering various purchases.

For me, there is no hurry, since, as the football ticket reads, I am a senior, eligible to watch the game in the student section, the S zone. Funny, thinking about it, even when I want to hurry, it is difficult, the masses a briar patch that snags me as I push forward. As soon as the gates open, and I am at the front of the line, I exchange my ticket for another with a specific row and number in which to sit, most of the time on the thirty-yard line.

I recall the day Michael made the high school football team. It was a turning point in his academic career. Now seizure free, he didn't have to worry about any outside stimuli that might have preceded a neurological reaction. The scar on his head was his trademark, he told me once. The distinct feature he was known for in the locker room.

Meanwhile, on the sidelines, I rubbed my scar and cheered him on. Michael was the starting quarterback, my favorite position. Unfortunately, I still had to worry about overheating and atmospheric stimulation that could start a seizure. These factors never kept me from attending the games. I loved it, and I love attending games today.

I did have an advantage over Michael when he was playing, though. I spoke with the beautiful Mary Grace, who had grown into an attractive young lady with a wonderful smile, and a quiet, almost meek, demeanor. She was even more attractive than when she was in middle school; having a slender curvaceous figure, light smooth skin, and a full face with high cheekbones. Better yet, her personality impressed me.

Mary Grace had no interest in popularity, refrained from complaining, and didn't compare herself to others to justify her actions. She had plans to be a nurse, and, she told me, nothing was going to get in her way. She was the real thing. Still is, I believe.

Anyway, she settled on the bleacher next to me, talking to me about her school day, and questioning about mine. We had a good time even when our school day was rough, and I felt proud sitting next to a pretty blonde with a great body. I never told her that, though.

Once inside the Beaver Stadium gate, I head towards a hotdog stand, a concrete booth with chip displays on the counter, and a big, blue board on the wall with all the menu items. There are several booths, each of which are somewhat hidden by the crowd, but I go to the one nearest to my seat and wait my turn.

• • •

I T IS hard to describe the magnitude of Beaver Stadium, the mere size of it. I'm pretty sure it holds 110 thousand fans. Every student here in State College who loves football, and who hasn't had the opportunity to experience the rush I get when I am in the third row of the student section, hasn't a clue of the power of Penn State spirit. There is nothing like it.

Initially, before the game starts, the most exciting thing for me is finding the seat, especially when I am right behind the players. I know I am thrilled when the staff walks up the ramp with me, and finds my place. At this point, the stadium isn't all that full. There is a faint smell of popcorn in the air, mixed with a hint of nachos and cheese. It takes a while for me to grow accustomed to the different odors.

Normally, I hand in the ticket two hours in advance, and once inside the stadium, I can't leave until the game is over. It works out perfectly, though, because I get to watch each team exercise, stretch, and practice different plays, the quarterback passing one ball to different receivers, the kicker repeatedly punting another ball across the field. The latest rap music blares, revving up the fans more and more as the hours pass, the replays of past games on the monitors instigating cheers.

About forty-five minutes before game time, Joe Paterno jogs out in his blue windbreaker and waves to the crowd, his notorious thick glasses accentuating his classic nose. He then claps as he talks with his assistant coaches on the sidelines. They jog back under the stadium, into the locker room after they have made their appearances.

Announcements are made, sponsors are acknowledged, and on occasion, other Penn State sports teams are called onto the field, recognized for an achievement, receiving an award. It is filler, of course, but nice to see nonetheless.

I get all riled up when I see the Penn State dancers kicking their legs up in the air in unison. They are dressed in short, dark blue sweaters and even shorter skirts. I check out each girl, observe her physique, and often think, *Come to papa!*

When the Blue Band marches out on the field in unison, the drummers, trombonists, trumpeters, and saxophonists forming the letters P, S, and U on the turf as they play the Alumni song, Hail to the Lion, I marvel, imagining the hours of practice that contribute to the band's synchronization. Their march usually brings in all the people, which means it is time to stand.

I really don't know why they call the benches in the student section seats, because you really don't sit at all during the five-hour game. Just about every student is either hopping up and down to encourage the Nittany Lions, screaming to distract the opposition and chanting negative phrases to taunt, or dancing and singing to music after we score.

When I think about the kind of person I am normally, sober and reserved, and the kind of person I am in the stands, a loud, antagonistic, emotional roller coaster, sometimes quaking out of anger and nervousness, I just have to shake my head. How can sports make me act like this?

The answer is easy. Penn State spirit. When I yell 'Go Joe!' or shout 'Joepa! Joepa!' or 'We are Penn State!' with thousands of people, even the bare-chested guys with shaggy, blue and white hair and painted faces, a sense of camaraderie washes over me, a sense of belonging. It puts a lump in my throat, and brings a smile to my face, an unfamiliar joy.

* * *

WHEN THE game is over and we have won, I am so wound up I have to take a deep breath. Several, actually. There is an ambulance out front of the stadium, and the lights are flashing, red lights rapidly flickering across my face, colorful bullets firing at my retinas. I begin to feel funny, hollow in my eyes, and sick to my stomach. "Shoot!" I mutter. "Here we go again." My auras always start at the most inopportune times.

I know I have to get down, on the ground as soon as possible. But where? Thousands of aggressive people are brushing against me, trying to pass me. There's no place for my preservation. Unless I can reach the group of parked campers, where all the tailgaters are. There are patches of grass there too. I walk with the crowd, still hoping I can make it.

Soon I see some grass, some tailgaters, but I know the electricity in my head is spreading, and I won't be able to hold out much longer. I see a few lounge chairs sitting ahead of me. Close by, two men with bloated guts are drinking beer, laughing loudly, and a boy is throwing a football in the air, and running to catch his own pass. I lay myself on the ground, right next to a camper. Someone is bound to find me.

Just as there was a time in my life when I dreamed or imagined certain situations in the color blue, I also had nightmares in shades of red. It only took minimal exposure to any color of red during my seizures to bring about a horrible, but plausible, nightmare. In my nightmares of red, I am falling eternally, only from the sky this time. I can't stop myself, gravity's mighty pull once again at work.

I have access to a red parachute, but it won't open, surges of fear pummeling my entire body. I search the backpack that tugs on my shoulders, looking for the cord that will trigger the parachute to unfold, to no avail.

A man in a red jumpsuit above me, also falling, yells at me, saying I am not listening. "You are doing it wrong, Chris. What's the matter with you?" I keep trying, but I miss the cord, the extension too limp.

The man has a devilish quality about him, glassy eyes, a contorted mouth with visible fangs, and fingers like talons. He aggressively claws the air, trying to grab my bag so I don't continue to drop, rapidly falling towards the earth. His hellish body is out of control, and the parachute he is floating under is starting to deflate, putting him in more danger than myself.

I see flocks of vultures soaring around us, avoiding us almost, but ready to feast on us if we perish. I also see exhaust lines from a plane in the distance. Why can't they help us?

I fall and fall and fall, the red clay earth approaching at an ever-increasing speed.

Next to the camper, my right arm is shaking hard, slamming against the aluminum siding. My mouth is touching the earth, red sod on my tongue. I grunt as I try to breathe, but all I get are brief whiffs of rubber from the rear tire. Spittle lines my lips. I feel a hand with long fingernails on my shoulder a moment later, and I hear myself yell out. One of the men with bloated guts hovers over me, the boy throwing the ball asking, "What's wrong with him?"

• • •

I AM A dead weight. A barbell. There is confusion all around me. The man is not a lifter, and has trouble maneuvering around me, unsure how to help me. I wonder why I am always found by the uninformed.

I feel as if I have been pelted by pieces of hail, my muscles bruised and strained by falls and solid crystals of weakness. The man says, "Take it easy, son. I'm here to help." The nerve of the guy! Telling me to take it easy. *Trade places with me for a few hours, and then shoot your mouth, buddy*, I think. *Can't you see me, here? I can't do a darn thing!*

I am now on my back, the worst position to be in when having a Grand Mal. For a moment, I had a surge of energy, and I got in a sitting position. I leaned on my wrists, which were trembling under the pressure, and I tried to lean forward. But my wrists buckled, and I fell sideways. Another surge of energy, and another failed attempt. I fell backwards, thus my current position.

I feel as if I am suffocating. I see bodies surrounding me, hear shuffling feet that sound like combat boots in action, constant motion. And I can't move. I get panicked. Incredibly panicked. I begin to whimper out of fear, my lips quivering. My body goes rigid, and I look from face to face, helpless and breathless.

• • •

IRONICALLY, THE same ambulance that started my seizure has come to save me; that's what the EMTs think, anyway. The vehicle is only a few feet away from me, and I dread what the people inside will soon do to me.

I want them to leave me be. Let me recover on my own. I don't want them to interfere. All my adult life, I have had to accept, if I am found by EMTs, they will want to involve medical staff at the nearest hospitals. I have had to accept they might have me lie down on a wooden pallet, and the possibility they might tie me down, wrapping me in buckles, even though I want to go home.

The lights are still flashing, and I have to wait. The wait is horrible.

• • •

I AM FORTUNATE. The EMTs don't buckle me down. I am wet and weak, though; my head is in pain, exploding like an active volcano. My body takes about forty-five minutes to rebound, and when I am fully functioning, I just want to get out of there. I sign the release forms, and begin towards Webster's bookstore. I have to lean on someone. Michael won't want to help, I don't think. He might be embarrassed.

It takes me longer to get there. I am still wobbly, and I am still breathing heavily. No big surprise. My rib cage was contracted for almost an hour. When I walk in, I see Sam wiping down the tables. I collapse onto a nearby chair.

The bookstore has grown, and I am happy about this. It means people are purchasing a lot of text. A number of new shelves full of books have been erected, and the lounging area has been rearranged. Sitting here, I think, *Chris! You are nuts! Go home!* But I have no one to go home to. I need someone to show me some sympathy. The exact same thing I normally don't want people to give me. Very contradictory, don't you think?

Sam doesn't turn around. He continues to scrub, his dreads falling around his face with every push of the dust rag. "We're gonna be closing soon, champ," he says, not realizing it is me.

"That a new tie dye shirt, Sam?" I say, still a bit breathless. "Very colorful."

He turns, looks at me more closely. "Chris, my friend. Sorry. I didn't know it was you." I tell him it's all right.

"You look like trash," he impulsively says. "What's up?"

"Just had a seizure. And I feel like trash."

"So, chap, why are you not home sleeping?"

"I thought about it, but I figured you would make me a free smoothie and lift my spirits."

He puts the rag in his pocket and walks behind the counter, pulls out his blender and scoops some ice cream. He then picks out a couple bananas and strawberries and mixes it with the ice cream. The blender roars as it softens the mixture. "When my boy was little. He was as stubborn as you are today. And if I didn't know better," he practically yells. "I'd think you were a mooch."

"Thanks," I say sarcastically, shaking my head. "I feel so much better."

"So. Tell me, was this seizure stress related?"

"I don't think so. The ambulance lights at the game did it, I think."

"I was just curious." He puts whip cream on my smoothie, and walks over to me. I grab the cup. "Considering how upset you've been with Michael."

I close my eyes, and put my head in my hands. "Yeah. He's been bothering me. But I don't think this seizure had anything to do with it."

$$\bullet \quad \bullet \quad \bullet$$

I AM BEAT this morning from the seizure at the game, and I almost stay in bed, but I get up. I make a decision I won't let my seizure hold me back. This is a decision I face daily. I feel horrible, but I arrive to the Chambers building for class on time. And I soak up some of the information given me.

My head is still aching; when I cough, laugh, or bend over, I cringe, an avalanche of pain plummeting over the dips in my skull. I deal with it, though. There are about twenty people surrounding me, all of them in individual seats wrapped around the room in a circle. There are people of different cultural backgrounds: Indian,

African American, and Caucasian mostly. Some Asian and African. The multicultural class consists of people in different programs outside my own. There are computers scattered against the walls, a table in the center of the room, and a chalkboard lined with children's crafts. I sit in the back, closest to the door, incredibly anxious to leave.

The whole class revs me up inside. I have a bad attitude. I am sick of it. The professors are intent on showing me how unfair life is for minorities. I get it. I understand people have feelings, have troubles as a result of others' behaviors, but I just can't believe the curriculum, the repeated emphasis on the fact that certain groups of people can't make it, that special treatment is necessary otherwise it is discrimination. Discrimination, my ass! I know discrimination exists, but using it as a crutch is not productive. How am I, as a counselor, supposed to empower clients, the whole point of counseling, if all I hear is clients will only be a success if they aren't discriminated against and are privileged?

I think every person is capable to be the best. Color, gender, and disability, in my case, may be setbacks, big setbacks, and they will make life hard, but, with help, I believe anyone can be a success. Instead, here I am, listening to some professors complain about their place in society, stereotyping people while preaching to do the opposite, playing the blame game.

I speak up. "It just seems like the minority in here are more hostile than the majority group, and the majority group . . ." I make quotation marks with my fingers. "Have been ripped apart for the past three hours." Someone objects to my comment, and I continue. "It would be one thing if we were talking about discrimination in the thirties, here."

I may be overly-sensitive because I am a minority, and I have succeeded despite my privilege, or lack thereof. I like the thought of having control over my life, and it eats me up when I hear people say otherwise. It also eats me up, because I know life is hard, and I don't need an educational institution to remind me of that. My daily life as a person with Epilepsy is reminder enough. Pain as a result of my seizures is reminder enough. Fear as a result of my seizures is reminder enough. Unwanted attention as a result of my seizures is reminder enough. Social and transportation setbacks as a result of my seizures are reminder enough. I know people with Epilepsy face difficulties, but no one hears us complaining, asking for special treatment.

When this class ends, I know my head will hurt worse than when I arrived. Three stinking hours of pessimism and promotion of division, generalizations and heated debate. But it has been good in one respect. The class has validated my self-confidence, and my confidence in others with Epilepsy.

• • •

To ALLEVIATE my annoyance, I head to the gym where I took my first lesson, where I am now learning Kali, the Filipino martial arts. I am finally participating in a sport of sorts. Now that I am involved in a physical activity, I think there is no better way to rid of my negative emotions than to use it to advance my proficiency.

The gym is in behind a pizza shop. It is a fairly large, open space with a boxing ring in the center, and a loft covered in wrestling mats where I have class Tuesdays and Thursdays. I take the class with about seven other students. I have been taking it a while, but I have a lot of room for improvement.

Michael had been taking the class with me. We always walked home together, congratulating each other on a win during our competitions, or empathizing with one another if either of us lost.

That was before Linda came along and stopped it. One day towards the end of the summer, three months after Linda and Michael met, Michael said to me, "Linda is afraid I will hurt myself. She wants me to stop fighting."

He explained that Linda appreciated intellect over physical brawn, that her mom raised her as an only child that way, and she'd been taught to resolve problems through discussion versus through any physical means.

You see, Michael informed me Linda hasn't always been attractive. At one point, she had numerous blemishes, and was pretty thick in the mid-section. She often came home crying because boys made fun of her, had hit her, or thrown rocks at her. At first, she responded in the same fashion, but it only made things worse. Only when she saw her mother address and successfully settle the situation with the other parents, did she realize it was better to be diplomatic about troubling circumstances. Thus, in her opinion, Michael told me, Linda felt he'd be more prone to act out physically if he continued training in the martial arts; especially Kali, since it is probably the most violent form out there.

"Well, what are you going to do?" I asked. "You love this, man. And it's not like you're training to beat up people who disagree with you!"

"I know, Chris, I know," he said. "But I think Linda might be the one. And I don't want to lose her."

"You do what you gotta do, man."

"Every time I went to karate class with you, she worried," Michael said. "She would rub my scar afterwards and say she didn't want me to have another one." *He used to love it in high school when the jocks complimented him on his scar*, I thought. *It's amazing what a girl will do to you.*

"Just think about it before you quit, " I said. "You've worked hard to get where you are." He had already made up his mind, though. He just wanted to hear what I had to say.

I think about this as I stretch my body, loosening my limbs to lift weights. I walk over to the weight room and get some twenty-pounders. Metal hits metal as a lifter places a heavy weight in its cradle. I sit down on a nearby bench and do some curls, determined to work through the burn. It is so easy to give in for me, but I have fortitude. I have always been a determined person, and I don't plan on changing in this respect.

I hear the bell ring in the background, sounding the end of a boxing match for a couple of men working out. The bell sounds frequently, and at times gets irritating when jumping around, sweating profusely, trying to concentrate in the sweltering heat.

I curl for a half hour, and move onto my karate moves. By the time I have finished practicing with my sparring sticks, and I have repeated my footwork matrix numerous times, my mind is clear. I feel revived and excited about my progress. Sort of proud, too. I can now go home and rest without resentful thoughts.

• • •

MOMENTS AFTER I have walked into my apartment and collapsed on the chair in my room, I hear what sounds like a herd of stampeding elephants, but what I have come to know as several people running up the stairwell to the third floor. Moments after that, I hear the herd snorting outside my door. And then in my living room. I forgot again that it is debate night.

I hear Linda say, "Okay. Tonight it's Aristotle." *Another discussion about reality*, I think to myself. *Thank God I did some research.*

"Yeah. Potentiality vs. actuality." Alex says. "I don't know if I buy it. And I bet you, Michael, that you can't win me over." More pessimism.

Michael looks at Alex, his brow furrowed. "The existence of anything has to have a cause, right?"

"According to Aristotle anyway!" John adds, punching his left fist into his right hand over and over again, as jittery as ever.

Ever the pacifist diplomat, Linda takes a sip of drink from one of my cups, root beer I think, then intervenes, "Now, now, boys. No need to be harsh." Her mom would be proud.

"Well, Michael starts. "There are four causes. The material cause. The efficient cause. The formal cause. And the final cause."

"True. True." Alex says, his forehead creased. "I'll give you that much." He continues, "But as far as I'm concerned, I'm not the cause of a life without a true family. It's not my fault my parents never were, and my grandparents are jerks!"

"And my mother caused me to run away from bullies. Not me," John adds. Everything is quiet. I'm telling you, it is an intense moment; time for my entrance. "Hey Chris!!" they all exclaim when they see me.

"Yo! You want to hear my thoughts?"

"Sure," they say in unison.

"Before I begin, I'd like to preface that you are looking at the concepts circumstantially, whereas I am looking at them materially." They all nod, encouraging me to keep talking.

"When I graduate," I announce, walking into the room. "My diploma will prove actuality." I go to the cupboard, get a cup of my own, and pour some root beer to quench my thirst.

"How so?" John wonders.

"It will exist on bond paper, proof of material cause. It will have been previously printed on the paper, proof of efficient cause. The Deans and President will have signed it and a stamp of completion will symbolize what it is, proof of formal cause. And it is the last formal document I'll receive from the university, proof of final cause."

"Impressive!" Linda squeals. "Very Impressive. Don't you think guys?"

"A very interesting analogy," Michael says, nodding.

John stops punching his hand. He seems at peace with what I've said. He wipes some sweat from his shiny forehead and smiles a little, grabs a Frito from a recently opened bag.

Alex rolls his eyes, but concedes, "Okay. You have a point."

• • •

 TONIGHT, THE same pillow that cradles my head turns into an adhesive. I wake up, and my head is a brick cemented by cotton mortar. I try to lift my head, but it doesn't move. Again, I am powerless. Depending on the night, the pillow won't let go for long periods of time. Other nights, I might only be stuck momentarily. Either way it is an awful experience.

I try to prop myself up, but I am unable. It is even worse when my mouth is inhaling the pillowcase. I try to spit the cloth from my mouth, and I get saliva everywhere. So, not only am I inhaling a pillowcase, I am inhaling a wet pillowcase. I sweat heavily, and I hear myself pant.

I am not exactly sure why my head won't move, but it only makes sense I have had a seizure that I was unaware of, and I am in my Postictal period, my motor skills in recovery. When I have the seizures at night, my nightmares are the most vivid, and probably more repetitive than a back-to-back, horror movie marathon.

I repeatedly dream about tornadoes, and how helpless I am. I run around looking for cover. I see through a window three dark funnel clouds ripping up the earth, houses split down the middle like tree trunks sawed in half. The window frame starts to shake, the wood beginning to peel, the paint chipping.

I can feel the force, even though the eye hasn't touched. I run around my apartment, look for a safe place in a closet under a stairwell. It is full. I run to my bed, to see if I can fit underneath. It is too low to the ground. I hear a voice yell, "Not there, Chris. You are gonna kill yourself! Over here!" At the same time, I hear another voice say, "There's no time to listen to him! Do what needs to be

done!" But I don't know what needs to be done. So I run throughout the apartment, looking under the kitchen table, and then the
cabinets under the sink. I even consider just lying on the ground,
my stomach and face against the floor, in the same position I am in
as I wait for my head to detach from my pillow.

Things start to fall, the ceiling fan, my lamps, the pictures I have
spent hours drawing. And then it happens. The window frame gives
in. The glass is thrust forward by the pressure, shattering everywhere. Shards surround me. Somehow I am still alive, and I look up
through what used to be a window, just an opening now making me
even more vulnerable.

I see debris thrown about. I see people and animals sucked up,
killed, and spit out as though Mother Nature doesn't like the taste
of them. I live through my dreams, but what makes them so horrible is that the twisters hover. They don't subside, and one wrong
move on my part could seal my demise.

Only when a lot of the cotton mortar disintegrates can I lift my
head up off the pillow, and I can sit up. I am fed up, and I ask God
why this won't end. No reply.

• • •

WHEN I don't hear a reply, it angers me. I punch my pillow. I sit
there in the dark, and ask myself out loud why I can't be normal.
Why can't I live a day without a darn physical problem? Sleep
through a night without excess brain activity? It just sucks so badly
sometimes, I become hopeless. It isn't fair! Why do I have to exist
like this?

At the same time, though it is hard to believe, I say, "Chris! Cut it out! Snap out of it!" I try to convince myself things could be worse. I've made it this far. I have lived through more pain and confusion than many have.

I think I am not dealt more than I can handle. I will make it. Tomorrow is a new day. Probably another day of auras. My seizures might get worse, but things are bound to improve. I have no clue what is the explanation for my condition, but I have Epilepsy for a reason. This statement is all I have to fall back on.

Hunched over, I sigh and shake my head. For whatever reason, I haven't gotten a sensible response from above for sixteen years. Figures.

• • •

DOESN'T LIFE just work like this, though? *Just when I am about to lose it*, I think, rolling my eyes, *something happens*. After sixteen years of trying to mix, match, and balance medicines, my neurologist calls me early this morning, just as I am drifting off, to tell me a new drug is out that, in his opinion, will control my seizures. Should I believe it and take it at face value, or brush the possibility aside? I've been let down by the medical community so often, I am apprehensive to trust anything doctors and nurses say. Believe me, I want to trust them. I do.

"So Chris. Are you still there?"

"Yeah. I'm here."

"Sorry to call so early, Chris. But I think there is a possibility we could take care of your seizures."

"No. It's all right. I'm up," I say, cradling the phone in the crux of my neck as I lean against the wall. "I had a rough night, a bad seizure, so this is good news."

"Well, as soon as you can get home, make an appointment, and come to the office."

"I'll do that." Maybe. I then turn the phone off and lay it on the ground, curl up under the covers, and fall asleep.

• • •

PART THREE:

YEAR TWO, SPRING SEMESTER, SEASONS END

I USUALLY ONLY get in a few hours of sleep after I recover my motor skills. I am exhausted, but I fear getting stuck again. So, once more, I don't get enough rest. Oh well. *I'll be dragging today*, I think. And early calls don't help enliven me any.

As I open my bedroom door on a Saturday morning following one of these episodes, I rub my eyes. I soon see Michael in the kitchen dressed only in boxers, making wonderful smelling pancakes. He has out syrup and butter, and my stomach mutters a desperate utterance.

"Hey Michael," I say, still rubbing the sleep out of my eyes. He has a grin on his face, an expression I usually see when he is thinking about his girlfriend.

"Hi."

I see a reflection from an unknown source on the wall, and I look around until I realize it is coming from Michael. He has a new earring. It is a gold stud, nothing special in my opinion, but a significant change for Michael. What an evil boy. I refrain from commenting on his change in style. I know he wants me to, but I decide not to talk about it, for it is his ear. Not mine. Besides that, I see someone else is here.

Linda walks out of Michael's room in a nighty. "Good morning, Chris." I try to flatten my hair, to make myself presentable. It is all over the place. I am shocked she is here at the apartment so early, but I don't show it. Had they slept with each other already? *I shouldn't really be surprised*, I think. *These days, it is so commonplace.*

"Morning," I reply.

Michael says to me, "Linda and I are going to visit her parents today." He places a stack of pancakes on a plate. "I haven't met them yet, Chris." I nod in acknowledgement. I think, *Wow, things are getting very serious between them now!* It sucks he is paying me less attention all the time. But, hey, that is his prerogative.

"Well," I say without sincerity. "I hope you have a good time."

"It should be interesting."

Michael and I usually went to a matinee on Saturdays, but that changed when Linda arrived, too. They go together now. I go by myself. Don't get me wrong, I enjoy my personal time; it is just hard letting go of traditions. I am a regimented person, routine-oriented, and any kind of change throws me off. Linda has brought so much change. I am having difficulty adjusting to college life without my best friend.

They sit down to eat with each other, converse as if I'm not in the room. She tells Michael about her parents. Uninterested, I go into the bathroom to take my medication and shower. I know it might sound funny, but I am feeling more and more alienated.

• • •

WHEN I feel neglected, I tend to retreat and draw. It is hard to explain, but I get this innate feeling that motivates me to create something, and, if I don't express myself, I get uncomfortable. Feelings of neglect and discomfort are counterproductive, so I decide to head out to Old Main again.

I was in a groove this past summer, but with a new set of classes scheduled, I was forced to reprioritize, to shift my focus back to my academic responsibilities. Everyone has to take a breather, though. At least I do. So, with that said, I collect my art supplies and head out, leaving Michael and Linda to their discussion over pancakes.

Over the past couple months I have collected a few photos I would like to duplicate in pastel, with my own personal twist, to be sure. I like drawing the elderly. I find it challenging to perfect wrinkles and folds in the skin, long intricate beards, and straw hats. So, I have some drawing options today.

On the way to Old Main, I observe a group of high school kids and their parents watch a tour guide as he walks backwards pointing to significant locales, and listen to him speak of the benefits associated with the university. They all shout, "We are . . . Penn State!!" The hopeful expressions on their faces remind me of how excited I was when I first took the tour with Michael.

Ignoring the tour guide, Michael said to me then, "We get through this school, man, and we are set."

I thoughtfully said, "Yeah. But it won't be easy."

"We want it bad, though," he said softly.

"You've got that right."

That conversation sticks out to me, because I can recall how academically driven Michael was. I haven't heard him talk of classes since he met Linda. But, you know, who am I to question his motivation?

Anyway, it is a fifteen-minute walk from White Course to Old Main, and it takes a lot of my energy to make it to my bench under the oaks without dropping my supplies. I only observe the group taking the tour briefly, and then I continue to my destination. I don't really know what my creativity will lead to this afternoon, but I'm sure it will amount to something. I won't be drawing a girl who reminds me of Mary Grace, but a stimulating person nonetheless.

• • •

ON MY way home, that foul taste in my mouth, the second kind of aura I experience, manifests itself behind my left molars. It really is bizarre, the sensations I sometimes get when I am in the early stage of a seizure. My mouth feels pasty, almost like peanut butter, and wet with bubbles. For some reason I grind my teeth and stare for a period.

I then stop in mid-stride, still grinding and staring. For a moment, I come to, and I try to speak. "Chri . . .ss." I slowly and intently say, consciously trying to overcome the looming seizure. "You . . . Uh." I lose my ability to speak. There is a glitch in the system upstairs. Then, alright again, I try once more, "Chri . . . ss. You. Can. Maaaa . . Uh . . . Make it." The sensation then leaves me. My mouth doesn't feel sticky anymore, and my molars are free of bubbles. I say out loud, "Thank you God."

Okay. I am back to myself for the time being. I look straight ahead, but I try not to stare at anything. Too much staring is sure to start up this episode again. I look at everything skittishly, the sidewalk for a minute, the sky a minute, the people around me for a minute, and then back to the sidewalk. I do this until I arrive back home.

• • •

THIS LAST episode is enough reason for me to make arrangements to see my doctor. I will have to go home and stay somewhere, so I call my parents to see if it would be all right to stay with them for a few days.

I haven't talked much about them, but they are a big part of my life. I know this is not the case for every young man, and I realize I've been fortunate enough to have my parents' support, throughout my childhood, my surgery, my high school years, and college career. I don't know if I got my critical thinking skills from them, but as a result of their pushing for the best, it is obvious they instilled in me their drive.

Unlike Michael, I didn't have constant concerns about being a sinner, and going to hell on a regular basis. Yes, I grew up in a religious household, as you may have gathered already in examining my thoughts. And, yes, I had that holy book, The Bible. But as long as I was wise, and made good decisions, I would not have to worry about anything. If I acted irresponsibly, my parents made clear, I would have to reap what I sowed. And this concept applied to me physically and spiritually.

Whereas Michael was threatened, I was encouraged to do the right thing, to live by The Book so that I could enjoy Christianity, and life in general for that matter. For a while they weren't into earrings and tattoos and wild hair, but with time, I can only guess, that changed. I imagine they thought preaching about physical appearance was second to pushing a lifestyle that included God.

As long as I tried to do the latter, I concluded, I was good to go. Even during my brief rebellious streak, when I didn't necessarily like my parents or anything they said, I deep down understood that their approach made sense. Since appearance was rarely an issue, I had no reason to pursue any form of body art. Thus, my current disinterest in permanent ink-jobs and holes in my body, and my incredulity about Michael's recent visit to the tattoo/piercing parlor. So he's in love. Why ruin his body?

Anyway, When I hear my Mom answer the phone, and she tells me she is putting me on speaker-phone so Dad can hear me, I imagine my parents in their piano room surrounded by pictures of jazz musicians playing instruments, next to the Grand, under the winding stairwell that leads to their loft above.

"I got a call from the doctor, and he gave me good news. I want to surprise you. Would it be alright if I catch a bus and visited a few days?"

Being the awesome son that I am, they have no problem with that.

• • •

I AM OFF on Fridays, so I schedule a visit to the doctor's office for the end of the week. On Thursday night, I arrive at the State College bus terminal and catch a Greyhound en-route to Harrisburg. The ride is not bad, about two hours.

For the first half hour I look out the bus window. The scenery is just incredible. My surroundings evolve as the thick, colorful woods and foliage bordering the mountain streams thins into flat, more developed land with very little vegetation. Meanwhile, the empty, windy roads turn into heavily traveled highways. Because I'm in the mountains, I enjoy observing the vast changes in climate, and it passes time away.

The time also goes by because I bring the book about the blind mountain climber. After the half hour of observation, I pull the novel from my travel bag. A couple weeks after I first skimmed through the novel at Barnes & Noble, I went back to the bookstore and bought it. Even though I find it difficult reading about the success of others, I get into this book for the remainder of the journey, and, before I know it, I am at the Harrisburg terminal.

My parents warmly greet me after I have gotten situated in their car, a sharp Jaguar. It's so great to see them. We exchange hugs and kisses, and then we settle on a restaurant where we will eat our dinner. We settle on a restaurant called Gullifty's, an interesting place with good food.

In Gullifty's, the eating area is poorly lit, sconces with an orange glow the only source of light. It is smoky, crowded, and loud. Several local bands perform on a stage in the downstairs bar, and it reverberates our booth. The waitresses are often strange, but the menu is great. It keeps us coming back.

After being seated by an eccentric hostess, while waiting for our dinners to arrive, my mother says, "You'll never guess who is working over at the neurology clinic."

"Yeah?" I say. "Who?"

"Mary Grace. You remember her. Right?" I think, *Do I ever!*

In a reserved tone, I say, "Yeah. I remember. She was good to me."

Sitting in the shaky booth, I am happy to be with my parents, and the news about Mary Grace makes it even better.

• • •

WHEN I show at the doctor's office, I walk to the front desk and sign the necessary paperwork, all the confidentiality crap. Handing the information to the secretary, I get sick to my stomach, thinking about my years as a constant patient. I look around. Sitting in the waiting room, other patients who probably know what I am talking about make noises, grunting, sighing, even yelling out, as a few seats away there is a man and woman with extensive neurological damage.

After waiting about a half hour longer than the actual scheduled appointment, I hear the door to the individual, examination rooms open. I hear a woman's voice say, "Chris?" The woman is Mary

Grace. She has on a white jacket, and is holding the clipboard with all the information I previously filled out. She is happy to see me, and smiles broadly.

I go through the regular protocol: the measurement of my height, the tracking of my weight. I usually don't care what people think of me, but because Mary Grace is the nurse following through with the protocol, I feel very self-conscious. I mean, I'm not fat or short, but I'm no skinny buff either. Of the two body types, I'd prefer the latter, especially when I am in the presence of someone significant.

She looks great, in my opinion, a sight for sore eyes. *She is definitely the ideal woman for me*, I think; Her long blond hair; her bright blue eyes; her smile; her slender body. She is as nice and wonderful as I recall from our days in high school.

Once we are in the examination room, she takes my blood pressure, which is probably higher because she is there, and she asks me how I've been. With a heavily beating heart, I shyly tell her I am nearing the end of grad school, and she congratulates me. I enjoy her touch on my arm and back, very nice. I ask her how things have been for her, and she tells me she loves being a nurse. Unfortunately, her work comes to a close. She documents my health status, and even though she probably shouldn't, she hugs me goodbye.

I see the doctor afterwards, which is much less exhilarating. I am happy he believes this new medicine will work, and I thankfully and willingly discuss my new options, but I don't enjoy the doctor near as much as the nurse.

• • •

JOSHUA HOLMES

A MONTH HAS passed since I have returned to my apartment at school. Everyday, I can see how in love Michael is. He won't stop talking about Linda! Linda said this. Linda said that. Linda did this. Linda did that. As annoying as it is, I know I'll probably do the same when I find my special someone.

Michael is an entirely different person. And I'm not just referring to his tattoo and earring. It is his overall demeanor; it changes on a whim if Linda wishes. Recently, he told me he has news, and I am curious to know which Michael I'll see then. He said he wants to tell me something over dinner at the cafeteria tonight. Before he does though, he told me he is going to walk Linda home.

I know this will take a while, so I go to the West Commons lobby early to watch some television, a game on the Big Ten Network possibly. There are some wooden benches in front of the TV, but I am uncertain whether or not I want to sit down. The seats are far from comfortable; there aren't any pillows. I don't want to sit if I can't have pillows, right? Right. So I stand. And I enjoy a game until it's time to head upstairs.

On the second floor now, I hand over the ID card I use to buy my meals to the lunch lady at the cafeteria entrance, and then take it back after it has been approved and twelve bucks has come out of my lion cash account. Wincing at the thought of such an amount decreasing my allotted spending, I enter through the door into the stuffy catering establishment.

I do not see Michael. For the moment, I sit down and wait. This place is a mad house! There are five main stations where kids hired by the school serve Chinese food, pizza, burgers and fries, and, my favorite, desserts like cake, cookies, and fresh Creamery ice cream.

• • •

As I wait, I think about the classes that have really helped me understand how people with and without disabilities reason and function. Human behavior intrigues me, and my program has a pretty thorough curriculum that, I think, helps you learn about it. This is what I need and like about the program, the substantial classes.

The Cedar Clinic, where I work for one of these classes, has its downfalls. The place hasn't been upgraded for ages. So, unfortunately, as a result, it is outdated, way too small, and, in my opinion, very uncomfortable.

I occasionally hear professors in my department discuss the impact of budgetary restraints. And at one point, considering the size of the university, I found their concerns hard to believe. But after laboring day and night at the clinic, hearing no mention of future upgrades, my doubts have dissipated, and I now accept a lack of funding is why my training ground isn't up to par.

In the clinic, there are about eight prison cell-like meeting rooms with large one-way mirrors covering the walls. Each room has two chairs in the center. One for the client. One for the counselor. In these cells, some additional décor includes a floor lamp, and a table with flowers, a microphone, a full tissue box for emotional clients, and a phone for emergencies (in case I have a seizure, for instance). Not a whole lot.

At the same time, I have good conversation with colleagues who are equally uncomfortable. As long as we are quiet behind closed doors, we can discuss our work, help each other explore counseling approaches, and refine the wording of our progress notes. And in regards to paperwork, I only have to put the Data Assessment Plans (DAPs) in a manila envelope, and walk down the hall to hand them in to the clinic coordinators. While the environment can be challenging, it has its benefits.

Working with clients in general for my practicum class is about as close for me to being a counselor as it will get at Penn State. This requires dedication to several hours of watching videos on old TVs in a hot, cramped room, and taking notes and completing self-evaluations in another, even smaller room. Depending on the number of referrals, I have carried a caseload of five clients at once.

During my sessions, I give my client direct eye contact. I dress appropriately, in a button-down shirt and slacks, and present myself in a professional manner, monitoring my posture and any non-verbals that might convey negative vibes.

While there is no room for error in this class, after my sessions with certain clients, I feel a sense of accomplishment. I am helping people who are hurting to sort through their problems, and when they have a revelation, or show signs of self-pride as a result of seeing things from multiple perspectives, it is rewarding. I have contributed to their happiness, and I go home happy as well.

• • •

GRAND MAL

J UST AS I am about to reflect on another influential class, Michael walks up behind me, taps me on my left shoulder, and then walks to my right. He does this to me all the time, so I know he is the culprit. Nevertheless, I am glad he is here, because I was about to give up on him.

Above all the chatter and gossip, Michael says, "Whaazuup homie!"

"Yo!" I reply, a bit anxious. "I'm good." I turn around and say with a smile, "So what's the story here, Mike. I've been waiting a while."

"Sorry. Busy with Linda."

"Get some food, meet me back here, and then you can tell me what you want me to know."

"Alright."

• • •

W HEN MICHAEL and I have sat down, we have to speak a little louder. All the undergrads are gossiping about petty things like who dumped who, who has a better haircut, or who got the most drunk the previous night. I still cannot get over how immature these kids are. *I'm sure glad I am not like that*, I think. I cringe when the group behind me erupts, loud streams of laughter filling my ears.

Our conversation begins lively and fun, as always. A lot of kidding and joking. Some light-hearted debate. Soon though, our joking and banter subsides and our discussion becomes sober.

"You know, Chris," Michael says, touching his ear where his highlighter usually resides, "I'm seriously considering dropping out of school." I immediately forget the obnoxious sounds around me. I stare at him in silence, my mouth open for at least three minutes.

"You've got to be kidding me, Michael!" I say. "Why the heck would you do that? You are nuts!" I am irate, shocked beyond measure.

"Cool it, bro. Let me finish," he says defensively, his lip starting to curl, his thick uni-brow starting to furrow. I can sense that the gossipers have turned their heads to listen in, to stare. I calm down and tell him to go on. "I'm in love, man. I don't want this school stuff anymore. I just want to be with Linda, on my own and not on campus."

"Well, I think it's pretty stupid if you want the truth." I am still in awe. "We are almost done here!"

"I thought you, of all people, would understand." He is thoroughly pissed. His voice is starting to rise. The employees at the dessert station now look at us. He pushes back his chair, picks up his tray, none of his food touched. "You know what Chris. I actually don't need your approval! I love her! She's got great parents! And she loves me!" He storms off, and everyone stares me down in a way that suggests they disapprove of me. I can almost hear them thinking, *What a dummy.*

I have a client to see in a few minutes, so I breathe deeply to cool off. I don't want to arrive at the Cedar Clinic disheveled. As I get up, I roll my eyes and think, *Considering the topic, that went pretty well.*

• • •

GRAND MAL

AT THE moment, despite my earlier, hostile discussion with Michael, things are going well. I just had a female client draw some personal conclusions. It was like a light bulb just lit up in her head. She realized what was holding her back (self-doubt, mostly), and how much power she has over her future. The first step to recovery.

Back in my room, I am rehearsing my introduction and confidentiality statement I have to reiterate with every new client. "As you know . . . everything we talk about stays in the counseling room unless I sense that you are going to hurt yourself or someone else . . . a child or an elderly adult." And the most embarrassing part. "And I have to tell you that I do have seizures. Are you uncomfortable with that?"

I am pondering over the last part when I hear the phone ring. I stop my rehearsal and think, *It's probably Mom and Dad checking to see how my day went.* To my surprise, it is Mary Grace. Having seen her recently, I have a renewed vision of her. And I like it.

"Hello?" I say, smiling to myself before she even responds.

"Hey Chris. It's Mary Grace." *Oh, cool,* I think.

"I know who it is. You didn't even have to say so." She laughs, and I see her in the doctor's office, in her white jacket, covering her mouth to maintain her professionalism.

"Well. Just calling to let you know the doctor talked to your insurance company, and you are good to go," she says. "You should be able to get your new med at the pharmacy now." It then gets quiet. As I told you earlier, I hate silence.

"You know Mary Grace . . ." More silence. "It was great seeing you again."

"Oh yeah." She says, a different tone in her voice. "Definitely. You too." I hear a chair squeak over the phone. Am I making her nervous? Is she looking around to see if her co-workers are watching? Or, probably the most likely answer, reaching for my records in the nearby file cabinet?

"Well," I say. "Thanks for the call. Talk to you later?"

"Yes. Will do."

• • •

ABOUT A week after Michael and I have our confrontational dinner, the Dave Matthews Band comes to town. Following our earlier discussion about my catching a ride with Linda and him to the concert, I reconsidered, and I am currently heading up Bigler Road by myself, a shortcut to the Bryce Jordan Center.

In my opinion, the Bryce Jordan Center is a great place to host special events. It is large and spacious, the round shape of the white structure conducive to large crowds. Inside, various vendors sell food at concession stands. Other vendors sell merchandise for the performing bands. And the atrium that circles out around the seating area is big enough so you can make it to your section in a timely manner.

Blue-collar families and students alike come together to share an entertaining evening at one of the best venues in all of Centre County. I get thrills just thinking about my time there. I don't know. I guess it's great for me because I am around a lot of different people again. Kind of like at the HUB and at Beaver Stadium.

Before I know it, I am close to the entrance. I am shivering because, no matter the season, the area just outside the Center remains chilly. A dry breeze just sucks the air out of me. Fortunately, I don't have to endure the chill too long, for the line to get inside moves quickly.

At the entrance, a security guard approaches me and says, "Spread your legs and raise your arms."

• • •

AFTER PASSING the security point, I hand my ticket to a lady dressed in a white, button down shirt, black slacks, a formal black vest, and a red bowtie. She tears off the stub, and hands the other half of the ticket back to me. She tells me to enjoy the show, and I tell her to have a good evening.

Inside the atrium, I buy some popcorn and a Pepsi, and then walk down to my seat. The Center is packed. I trip over a few people in the process of getting to my seat, but I get there and situate myself in a way so that I can place my food and drink out of harm's way.

There is a man in front of me, dressed in a tie-dye shirt (similar to Sam's) that says 'Legalize Hemp'. He has a long mullet and spectacles comparable to those worn by John Lennon. He leans back in my direction and says with a toothless smirk, "I've seen these guys five times! Gone to 'most every concert! You?" His breath reeks of alcohol. He is clearly intoxicated, and I am not interested in speaking with him. He looks at me, pushes a doobie in his mouth, and waits for a response.

I act as if I didn't hear him, turn away and pick up my soda. I know the types of people who can come to see the Dave Matthews Band. There are the social weed smokers, the druggies, and the deadheads. Mr. Mullet seems to be a drunk deadhead. I'm not saying there aren't classy people who come to the Bryce Jordan Center for some contemporary jazz, but the carefree nature of the music, and the lyrics about the joys of getting high often brings out the craziest of people (not to mention a select few who enjoy surfing the crowds, exposing their nude bodies to the world). I smile at this thought, as I remember when it happened a few years back at the Hershey Park stadium.

The concert hasn't even begun, but the air is thick with smoke; the illegal drug a dark fog floating around me. It is stuffy, and the fog makes me claustrophobic, but I have gone through this before. I know what the concerts are like. I have been to six of them. My favorite band's gigs have always made my claustrophobia go away. For an hour and a half, I wait for Dave, Leroi, Boyd, Carter, and Stefan to walk on stage. I am surprised the ushers haven't approached Mr. Mullet.

• • •

WHEN THE lights dim, the vapor seems to fade. The crowd roars. In the dark, we all hear the smooth saxophone sound. The bass guitar follows a short, horn solo. Still in the black, the violin and drums come to life. And finally, I recognize Dave Matthews is strumming his acoustic guitar. In unison, they open the concert with their famous song, 'Crash'. The moment Dave begins to sing, the stage lights flash on, and the crowd roars even louder.

On either side of me, young couples are kissing, hugging, and dancing with one another. All around, other people in the audience are holding up cigarette lighters, giving a candlelight ceremony effect.

I begin to sing, "I'll be your Dixie chicken if you'll be my Tennessee lamb, and we can walk together down in Dixieland. Crash into me." A girl behind me rubs my shoulders, and I look back thinking, *What the heck?* She is wearing a bandanna over dark French braided hair, a halter-top, and very short shorts. She says, "Crash into me, baby." And she sticks out her tongue. I shake my head, and turn around. First it was Mr. Mullet, and now The Tongue. What an experience.

Again, though, Dave and the band overwhelm me, and I continue to have a great time. They start to jam, which they have long been known for, and their ability to improvise their songs on a whim is unbelievable. The keyboardist starts playing a cover band song, 'Super Freak', and they all join in with their individual instruments to build the crescendo.

Leroi, the saxophonist, is a big guy who plays with sunglasses and a straight face. Carter on the other hand drums with a big smile on his face. Boyd is constantly sliding his rod over the violin strings; his eyebrows lifted high, his smile spread wide. Dave and Stefan sing and play with intensity, and dance while they perform, moving their feet back and forth.

At the peak of the song, the strobes start to sparkle. Green, red, and blue lights flicker on and off with each beat. The colorful display continues for a long time, and the music overwhelms me, filling me with that happiness I feel at the football games. The display grows more and more elaborate, like fireworks during a celebration, until the song slows down and eventually comes to a close.

I stand for three hours as they play old and new tunes, and Mr. Mullet and The Tongue leave me be. I haven't stood for three hours straight since football season, but I'm running on adrenaline. I am at Penn State, taking a break from my work, listening to my all-time, favorite band while feasting on junk food. It doesn't get much better than this. The air is thicker with smoke now, but I am used to it. I knew I would get over it, and time passes quickly. I tap my fingers on the back of the chair in front of me, and sway to the music.

Before I know it, the concert is over, and it is time to stop dancing. Dave and the band close with their usual song, 'Stay', and he thanks everyone for coming out. He says, "See you all next year. Be good to one another, you hear?" And the stage goes dark.

I think, *Man! Once again, they surpassed my expectations!*

•   •   •

WALKING HOME, I think about Michael and Linda; whether or not they enjoyed the music or made out the whole time like the other couples around me. I wonder what my night with them would have been like. I didn't have a seizure, a stoned deadhead said hello, and a girl hit on me. Not that that's a bad thing. I just wasn't hanging with friends. For a moment, the thought makes me angry. But I again tell myself I am being unreasonable.

If I were to ask Michael and Linda about it, they both might get defensive. Unfortunately, I tend to ask questions in the wrong way. I am often misunderstood. I inquire about things most people don't like to discuss. It's not my fault I want to find explanations.

Speaking of finding things, I sometimes have difficulty finding my way home in the dark. I have to ask people where to go. Tonight, though, I know where I am. I cross University Drive, which is barricaded, pass the Bursars Office to my left, as well as the Wagner Building (a.k.a. the ROTC building). Orange cones and orange netting line the sidewalks to protect the kids from hazardous areas under construction. So many students are walking home to their dorms.

I, on the other hand, am going to White Course. So I stroll beyond all the dorms. I head towards the enormous walkway crossing North Atherton Road, where Michael claimed he wasn't winded from the hike. I won't deny it, tonight. I am exhausted. And I have to get up early tomorrow for my individual supervision meeting concerning my clients at the Cedar Clinic.

When I reach my apartment, I might read a while to settle myself down, to clear my head of all the sights and sounds of the concert. I will not watch TV, though. I'll have a chance to do that just after daybreak, as it is protocol to view a video of my counseling session with my supervisor.

• • •

I DO READ when I get home, but I fail to notice that the red light on my phone is flashing, that I obviously have a new message.

I accidentally close my eyes, and doze off on my bed with my glasses on. And as with the lights from the ambulance at the game, the flashing light on my phone throws me into a seizure. Right now, the intensity of my seizure is pulsating.

Because I just went to the Dave Matthews Band concert, my mind is filled to the brim with images of dancers, singers, instrumentalists, and lovers. Not to mention visuals of the entire auditorium blanketed with a suffocating cloud of weed and apparitions holding lighters in the air. These are normal images, but I am about to see a distorted version of them I wouldn't wish on anyone.

My brain currents are presently at full throttle, and I am heading into a delusional state. In this state, I am entering the Bryce Jordan Center again, falling soon after, and hitting my head. I am sweating from my efforts to breath, and I silently cry. My lifeless body is pinned under the Center's smoky coating. I can't lift my head, move my arms or legs, or make the dancers and singers aware of my horrible condition. Like a fireworks display gone awry, the stage lights are intensely flashing in my face every color imaginable.

When those people nearby do see me, they all laugh. Mr. Mullet scoffs, says, "Look at him. It is his fault he hurt himself. He shouldn't have been tapping his fingers on my chair!!" I begin to wail. I want to say, "Get away from me!" But all I can do is loudly grunt and attempt to grab at the air. I am so scared.

The Tongue bends over me, and says, "Yeah. He wouldn't be my Dixie Chicken either!" I see ushers with small bodies and big heads running down the stairs to my aisle. Behind them, I see Dave,

Leroi, Stefan, Carter, and Boyd making faces at me. Then they laugh and laugh and laugh. My favorite band. All of them making fun of me.

My dream is torture. My sleep is torture. My seizure is torture.

• • •

MY RESTLESSNESS makes getting up less torturous, though. Remember Mrs. Patterson? The sometimes aggressive, but mostly caring, bouncy-haired professor with whom I had difficulty my first semester? In my second year, she is my practicum supervisor. We get along well now, and I don't have to worry about her piercing eyes boring into me near as much.

When I arrive at Mrs. Patterson's office, I can see from the hall that she is moving a few pieces of paper (Imagine! Only three papers!) off of her file cabinets, putting them on her empty desk so that the television and cassette player will fit on top of the metal surface.

I tap on the door, which is only half open, and she tells me to come in. I sit in that once dreaded seat. It isn't quite as scary as it used to be. It helps that I'm tired, and that sitting in any chair sounds good to me.

After Mrs. Patterson inserts the cassette, she soberly asks me what I thought about my session with my client.

"I think it really went well," I say with a nod. "Really well."

On the television, I look so much more reserved than I feel. I have my legs tucked under my seat because I really want to bounce my foot when speaking with my client, and I have my hands folded because I know I will start tapping my shoes if I don't. Yet it all looks so natural!

My questions don't sound near as bad as I thought, either. My client's reactions are very positive. Everything about the session makes me feel better about myself. I might just turn out to be a good counselor!

When we are done watching the video, Mrs. Patterson wipes a few dust particles that fall out of the cassette player (no kidding), and then we discuss the plan for my next session. She advises me not to problem solve, but rather let the client take the session where he wants it to go. I assure her I will, and she says, "You've come a long way."

• • •

I GUESS I have come a long way. I'm proud of myself! My hard work is paying off. But I don't know if I can say the same thing about my best friend. Michael has gone somewhere, too, but not in the same way. His Dad's training has disintegrated. Michael has almost stopped working on his homework all together, and he has stopped participating in his debate club.

John and Alex are standing outside my apartment door to see if Michael and Linda are ready for a debate. Both Michael and Linda are out and Michael recently told me he was going to quit the group meetings. Alex's forehead is creased like you wouldn't believe, and his pudgy fingers are in the air, just emphasizing something I didn't hear. John's forehead has a nice white highlight in which I can see a distorted version of myself (when he comes to a momentary standstill, that is), and he is annoyed that I didn't open the door sooner.

I don't want to tell them that their intellectual colleagues have no desire to participate in their explorations of philosophy any longer, yet I have to say something. I don't want them to feel rejected as I frequently did growing up, so I say, "Guys, I'm sorry to break the bad news, but Michael and Linda will be busy with other things from now on."

I imagine how much John and Alex will miss their weekly gatherings around that pitiful table, the camaraderie and banter as they tried to get comfortable on the hard seats. Yeah, they will have a hard time walking away from the experience.

It was a time when Alex could let off steam about his nasty and neglectful Grandparents, and express his desire for a Dad, a "real" role model. This time also allowed John to stay in the present, without worries of being attacked.

While I did not really enjoy the banter, I enjoyed some of the theory, and was learning more about how my friends, yes, my friends now, thought. I will miss the experience, too. If for no other reason, I was becoming more open to new ideas. I now know that it is important to listen, even if I disagree, and this philosophy falls in line with that of my counseling program.

"What?" they say simultaneously. "How can that be true?"

"They are finished with the club." They turn to leave, shaking their heads.

"I know," I agree, shaking my own head. "It's sad."

• • •

To MY dismay, I am not aware of the moving date, when Michael has to be out of his room. So, initially, I am annoyed. And, to top it off, I still do not approve of his decision to leave school. But again, my opinion doesn't mean much at this point.

Michael and Linda start cleaning early in the morning, too early for me, and I do not know why they can't wait. I hear a familiar sound, the large golden dolly from the community center vestibule crashing against the sides of the doorway. Once in our kitchen, the squeaky wheels screech to a halt, and, still in bed, I say to myself, "For crying out loud. Am I ever going to get a solid sleep?"

Perhaps when I graduate, when I'm too tired to do anything but close my eyes! I guess I'll find out when I get there. In the meantime, I know complaining isn't going to put me back to sleep. So I get up. I recognize that I will be better off getting my endorphins going. Once again, in my classic Christopher fashion, I dunk my head in the sink and push my matted hair back into an acceptable position. "Morning," I say to the busy couple, yawning. "You really know how to give a nice wake up call."

"Sorry, Chris," Linda says, peeking from behind Michael. *What's up with all this peeking?* I think. *Are we playing hide and seek here?*

"It's alright," I lie. "So where do we begin?"

"Well you could help us with the boxes. They need folded and taped so we can start putting my things inside." Michael points to the boxes in the corner, and hands me the tape. The boxes are right next to my art supplies. "You might want to brush your teeth, too. I don't want you to knock us out on moving day!" We laugh a little, which is a nice change from the yelling he gave me before the Dave Matthews Band concert.

The living room is bright today; the blinds pulled all the way up. The sun is shining, and I have to squint for a while. I think about the night Michael and I stood before the same window talking about the pitiful ditch by the bus stop. It really wasn't all that long ago. I think about doing our homework in silence, and throwing the foam football around while watching the Steelers.

I then think about the day Michael first brought Linda to our apartment, how the door was locked. And when he smirked those goofy smirks while cooking for her. When she walked out of his room in a nighty, my hair a crazy mess.

"Are you going to be taking the television, Michael?" I ask, hoping he won't.

"I'd like to," he replies, itching his ear. "Are you all right with that? Because I was going to pay you the amount you put towards it." While it is hard to part with such a nice piece of technology, I am okay with it. I have a television in my room.

"Yeah," I say. "That'll work."

Before we start carrying the boxes down to a rented truck, I go to the bathroom and thoroughly scrub my teeth. While I had the urge to make my friend suffer a whiff, a sign of a true friend, I have mercy on him. No use leaving a sour taste in his mouth.

It takes several trips up and down the elevator to finish the move. And the move leaves its mark. That's for sure. The dolly has destroyed my doorway, the doorframe nicked and sliced, and I can pretty much forget getting back my initial down payment. Very disappointing.

Even more disappointing, though, is the fact that my best friend will be gone at the end of the day. For good? I don't know. I hope not. But things don't look too promising. Michael just told me he'll be proposing very soon. A good indicator.

Let me clarify, though, that I feel the time I spent alone helped me grow. I'm more independent. At one point, I needed Michael by my side just to get by. No longer. I will remain friends with John and Alex. I will continue going to karate. I'll deal with my Epilepsy with assistance from above, and I'll finish up my degree a stronger person.

After I put the last box away in the back of the truck, I turn to Michael and Linda. I hug them, and look at Michael. "I'm going to miss you."

"Yeah. Well don't get all sappy," he says, patting me on the back. "We'll be around."

● ● ●

PART FOUR:

SPRING AND SUMMER SEMESTER, SEASON FINALE

I DECIDE NOT to get emotional about Michael and Linda's departure. My emotions have to be saved for other things. After all, I have an internship to get ready for. Perhaps one at the Office of Rehabilitation Therapy, the agency my department wants every student to get into so they can maintain their almost 100 percent job placement success rate.

I have to make the calls to all the ORT county administrators in the state for possible interviews, the calls to Pennsylvania's Civil Service office so I'm on "The List". The list that supposedly helps me and tells each county I'm available for a position. The list that can, I've heard, also come back to bite me in the rear. The list some administrators can tell me I'm not on if I have a disability like Epilepsy, even if I am.

Do I settle for an unpaid internship with mentoring responsibilities at a smaller agency, or work for a possibly discriminatory government agency counseling, shuffling papers, and pushing as many people as likely into employment? A tough question that is emotionally challenging.

So I have other things than my friend leaving to think about. I'm putting all options on the table. And I'll see soon what happens.

• • •

THE SPRING semester is moving along slowly, because ORT has bitten me in the rear over and over and over again, just as predicted. And sure enough, my transportation problem has provided the state agency an excuse to eliminate any professional opportunities I have earned.

I have gone to ten different interviews, all of which I did well, and been turned down. Talk about a major blow to my ego, and an incredibly disheartening series of events. By now, all my friends from the original group are gone, either in their internship or working full-time. And I am still waiting with no opportunities in sight.

I call my parents every night to vent. I sort of feel bad about it. They shouldn't have to worry about me after a hard day's work. They have their own issues to deal with. Who else do I have to talk to, though? Well, I guess there is Sam. Yeah. Now that I think about it, I do have Sam.

• • •

"OK SAM. So here's the deal," I say. "I'm still unemployed with no sign of anything in sight. And I am stressing like you wouldn't believe."

"You know, Chris. Don't be in such a hurry. Waiting isn't such a bad thing."

Observing the new pictures on the walls in the bookstore, and then the new bookshelves to be filled, I say, "That's easy for you to say."

Staring at me intensely, he replies, "I'm an old man, chap. Look at me. I lost a wife ages ago over money. I longed for but never had a son. I have a bum leg. And dreads that look a hundred years old. Don't tell me I don't know about time."

This shuts me up. He's right. "Sorry."

"It's fine. Just remember that patience is a virtue." Cliché, but true I guess. And then a broad smile crosses his face. "On a different topic. I've noticed that you have been keeping an eye on the artwork on my walls. I know you are a great artist and I think it's about time you give a show."

"Oh, Sam. Would you let me?" I look at the pictures again, more intensely. I am trying to visualize my drawings in certain positions along the wall. The mildewy smell of used books and the odor of coffee wafting from a nearby table does not distract me. I'm too excited by the thought of my own show.

Smiling what feels like an evil smile, he says, "In time, son. Very soon that wall will be yours to use."

I pick up a book and purchase it. *In time*, I think. *Very funny.*

• • •

I TAKE THE book I bought at Webster's to a secret garden I found in front of the Alumni Hall just recently. The garden is hidden behind a white gazebo wrapped in the brown and maroon leaves of two Japanese Maples. A narrow pathway covered in silt opens into a shady area with wraparound benches. Ready for a nice read, I take a seat and cross my legs. At my feet, several slate stones accentuate a small, man-made pond where tiny ducklings float on the surface and a turtle's head peeks through the water ripples. This little world is so beautiful it is surreal, and a place so remote I could stay here forever.

Reading forever. Huh. That's a thought. And it's not like I don't have the time. Yeah, I have some papers to write for a few classes, but other than that . . . Nothing but time. Just waiting for an internship opportunity to hop on.

Since the nonfiction novel about the blind mountain climber was good, I bought another nonfiction novel; only this one is about a guy with quadriplegia who paints with his mouth. The story is right up there with the story of an artist/novelist with severe Cerebral Palsy who goes from poor boy to nationally acclaimed painter and author in *My Left Foot*.

I look at my left foot. It makes me think about my karate class, how much I have improved. How my body is doing more than I ever thought possible. And how, surprisingly, I am seizing less. I will be learning new kicking techniques this week. I have been kicking punching bags that my opponent holds up, but from what I understand, I will be kicking my opponents without punching bags, and with very little protection; maybe gloves and a mask at most. This thought peps me up.

A nice breeze cools my warm hands, and the book's pages between my fingers rustle quietly. I hear a splash in the water, and I assume the turtle is ducking beneath the surface. While I could stay here for many more hours, I fold the corner of the last page I've read, close my book, and bow out of the secret garden, back into the real world.

• • •

IN THE real world I have spent a lot of time focusing on the inconvenience of my seizures, and of waiting. I haven't focused on one positive thing. Ever since I started taking the new medicine, my seizures have decreased substantially. And my visit to the neurologist, and correspondence with Mary Grace, has led to a less distracting lifestyle. These are good things. Necessary things, in my opinion. Why, you ask? Because I don't know if I could take unemployment and constant seizing at once. It just might break my will.

Despite yelling at God, at my lowest moment He opened a door and made His presence so clear. He had the woman I've had a crush on my entire life take care of my prescriptions. Too coincidental to be fate. I haven't been given more than I can handle. Given enough, though, that my "human resiliency", a term frequently used in the counseling field, was and continues to be necessary. I persist in hopes that He will shine through.

For some reason, as I walk past the Alumni Hall, approach Pollock Road, and the garden disappears, I feel rejuvenated. I sense that there is something good on the horizon.

• • •

MY PREMONITION may prove true today, twenty-four hours after I have visited the garden. My internship woes could be wiped away. Just recently, I called a friend of my advisor's, a doctor currently working as a counselor at a job placement agency called CareerForce. Over the phone, she said she would give me an internship if I give her a good interview.

So I am walking up Allen Street at the moment. I am dressed in a powder blue button-down shirt, a navy suit coat, navy slacks, and a navy blue and powder blue striped tie. My Adam's apple is bulging out of my neck, which is a bit uncomfortable, but other than that, I feel great. My head is held high, my dark hair slicked back. I take a deep breath, and I smell my cologne, my skin exuding a nice aroma.

I look at my reflection in the windows of the surrounding stores to make sure I look handsome, and I smile, giving myself a thumbs up. I am almost at Panera Bread, where I made arrangements to meet with the doctor. Just above my cologne, I can smell sandwiches and soup, a great combination.

The doctor told me she would be in a plaid shirt and pants, that her hair is short and dark. I see so many women with dark hair sitting at small tables, circular booths, and couches. While I am excited, I momentarily get worried. What if I don't find her? But my concerns go away when I see a lady in the corner wave at me. She is wearing an open, black sweater over her plaid button-down. No wonder I missed her!

I walk over to her and stick my hand out for a shake. "Hello Dr. Webber. I am Chris."

• • •

I HAVE ALMOST every interview question and response out there memorized. As I sit down, I quietly recite my opening, and hope for easy queries. My heart is beating fast, and I am shaking inside. When the questions are basic, mainly pertaining to my counseling experience, and the requirements to fulfill my internship, I relax.

However, I must say the lack of affect in her voice confuses me. Is she bored? Am I coming across confident enough? An hour passes, and as the clock ticks, I overcome my self-doubt and make an assumption; that she senses I am reliable. And before I know it, Dr. Webber says, "As far as I'm concerned, you can start tomorrow."

I say, "Dr. Webber, thank you so much. You have no idea how grateful I am."

"No problem," she replies, smiling. "You should have called me sooner!"

• • •

WHEN I step into the CareerForce office for the first time, I am so pleased. It is quiet, open and airy, a pleasant atmosphere. Every employee is talking softly either in their cubicles, near the printer, or at the front desk. Each one seems to be enjoying their colleague's company and assistance. Some of them stop what they are doing to welcome me, and I tell them a little bit about myself, to break the ice.

When they all hear that I am completing my master's degree at Penn State, they congratulate me, and I smile appreciatively. I especially enjoy the secretaries. They seem as if they were born to meet and greet.

One secretary in particular, Sally her name is, reminds me of Jenny on *Forrest Gump*, the blond hippy in a long dress who carried a guitar around after joining the Black Panthers. While Sally isn't a Black Panther member and isn't carrying a guitar, she does have Jenny's golden eyes, a plain, full-length dress, and loose, scraggly hair held in place by a red bandanna. Her voice is so fluid, and she pats my back when she says she looks forward to working with me.

Dr. Webber says, "Well, Chris. Now that you have met some of the employees, I'll show you around, and then we can talk some more."

In the front area, there are about twelve computer terminals for unemployed individuals to job search. The people sitting before the keyboards are unkempt, dressed in torn clothing and covered in long, ratty hair. All their faces are tense as they concentrate on the agency's database. And they seem to know what they are doing, almost as if they visit the office regularly.

Dr. Webber walks me down a hall. She walks with intensity, as if she's on a mission. To some extent, she is. I can tell she is excited, but she maintains a solemn expression. She is kind but serious. I later learn that this is just her personality.

She points to a room on my left with more computers, where I assume the career counselors teach certain classes. Just opposite the computer room is a large conference room. Any number of meetings could be held here. Moving on, she points to three small rooms that all contain a tiny table, a chair, and a phone. She says, "Customers who need to make cold calls to employers can use these rooms."

The tour continues, and even though I've been in several offices, I'm still interested. After all, I'll be working here for the next three months. So, I am best off learning my way around immediately. Dr. Webber briefly shows me the last conference room, the bathroom location, and the small kitchen/eating area. In the corner of the eating area, I see a candy machine, where I can buy candy for a quarter. I smile and think, *Yes!*

Dr. Webber must sense my delight, for she adds, "By the way, there's a vending machine around the corner." I think, *Yes, Yes, Yes!*

• • •

STANDING WITH my student clients at Penn Tech, I say, "Yes. I think you will do well if you come here for school." Dr. Webber nods in agreement, a slight smile on her face. The technical school is small in comparison to Penn State University, but I have never seen a technical school so nice and spread out. In my opinion, the layout is impressive. Perfect for students who have adjustment issues. The college does not have numerous dorms that take up space, but rather a few apartment complexes that house everyone on campus. We all begin towards one of the complexes.

"Maybe," one of the older girls says. Jane, a chubby redhead with hazel eyes and bad teeth, is challenged both mentally and physically. She has depression, and walks with a limp; her demeanor always solemn, her one leg pretty atrophied. Her condition has prevented her from excelling in high school, which is why she was referred to Dr. Webber's program. She might have some impairments, but I believe she has real potential. "Maybe not," she adds.

While I believe in her, I have to be realistic too. She has multiple hurdles to jump over in order to reach some form of success, of normalcy or independence. Unlike other students her age, Jane will have to work twice as hard to achieve half of what "ordinary" kids are capable of; any chance of social play limited just to keep up academically. As you may have gathered by now, I'm an exception to the rule. And for all I know, she could be too.

The entrance to the complex is rustic, long shadows extending from a red, brick archway with an open black, cast iron fence. I feel like I am at a baseball game, ready to hand in a ticket so I can go inside to find my seat. I even have to walk by a nice patch of green grass with four white stones at the patches' edges that could pass for bases.

I walk in last place; behind the students who are absorbed by the information the tour guide is giving us. While I am excited for the students, I again think of the time Michael and I took the tour. We were absorbed, and had high hopes, yet it wasn't enough for my friend. I hope my clients' interest is an indicator of an uninterrupted, bright educational future.

The apartment setup is different but nice. Two students to a bedroom. Of course, I like my apartment better, but that's just me. The parents of the other students on the tour are absolutely thrilled for their sons and daughters who plan to attend in a few months. It is a day of bonding. And to think a prospective bedroom could bring a family together.

I feel as if this trip has improved my relationships with my clients. I think speaking to them all on their level gets rid of the intimidation factor. Yeah. I remember when I thought some of my teachers in school were arrogant, and I don't want to come across that way now.

Jerry, a young man of sixteen with blonde hair, brown eyes, and multiple piercings in the ears digs his hands deep in his pockets, sags his shoulders in despair, and says, "I dunno man. I want to do it. I been accepted, but I failed 'da test.'" Jerry has a learning disability. He comes from a low-income family, and he hasn't been encouraged all that much. I know he can get through this school with a lot of tutoring, and I plan on pushing him hard, going the extra mile to motivate him.

I don't plan to push him too hard, however, for I know what it is like to have others encourage me with good intent, but not acknowledge the impact a condition can have on my ability to perform. I understand how frustrating it can be, and I won't excessively nag him about what I think he can do, if he doesn't believe it himself. Subtlety is key, and I can counsel him in this manner.

I have been doing this for two months now, counseling several students like Jane and Jerry. I enjoy working with the lost youth as opposed to the stubborn college students I probed in my practicum, and I hope, one day, to find a job in youth counseling.

• • •

THINKING ABOUT my hopes for a job in this field back at my apartment one night, I say a silent prayer, asking for a job opportunity. He gave me my internship; now I need employment.

I sit on the couch in the stillness after talking to God, and look at the wall. Against the wall, there is a box in which I see a rolled up piece of paper bent at the edges. I am curious as to what it is, and I get up to retrieve it.

To my surprise, the decrepit piece of paper holds the picture Michael drew for me when we were boys, the picture of Mary Grace in the color blue, the angel flying in a navy sky, descending into cobalt clouds. What a shock. I look at it, drifting off to a distant place when life was simple. All those memories.

I am so pleased that I have something that I can hold onto, something that reminds me of Michael. I look at it for a while longer, soaking up the distorted image of my favorite nurse. His depiction of her is classic. Just awesome.

I place the drawing in my lap and close my eyes again. I let my worries about finding a permanent job leave my mind, leave them to God, and I turn my thoughts towards graduation. I'm unsure about many things in my future, but I am certain that He will take care of them, and that I want Michael and Mary Grace at my commencement.

● ● ●

IT IS early at the office, and nobody in the resource area has come to me for assistance on the computers, so I am looking at a letter the Jostens Company recently sent me. The letter is a reminder that commencement is drawing near, and it is about time that I buy graduation announcements, custom seal note cards, and certificates of appreciation as the momentous day approaches.

I am counting the number of weeks I have left of my internship at CareerForce when a heavyset middle-aged lady with premature wrinkles, a bulbous nose, and a big gap between her two front teeth walks up to my desk.

"Ya work 'ere?" I nod and think, *As an intern anyway*. I started not too long ago in the computer area, but I have taken over many of the customer service responsibilities. It's been interesting.

"Yeah. How can I help you?" On the form she hands me, I see her name is Barbie. Let me tell you. This lady looks nothing like Mattel's famous doll.

"Well. I jus' quit my job. The boss was a bastard." *Oh. Good excuse*, I think.

"So what field are you interested in?" I hope she has a special interest, but I don't expect it, as so many that have come in just want money, no matter the source or at what cost.

Barbie laughs nervously, her crow's feet extended in every direction. "I'm desperate, son. Anything will work really."

Inside, I wish now that Sally, the secretary, had a guitar, and would entertain this woman. I have no problem with helping Barbie, but considering Sally is around her age, grew up in her era, and has been in customer service a lot longer, both ladies would bond more quickly, I'm sure. Barbie would listen to Sally.

I try not to push the issue, but I tell Barbie it is important to find a job that best suits her as a person, that it will make the job search process easier if she knows what area of work she wants to pursue, and if she has some realistic goals. I add, "Think about it a minute, and then come get me." She nods.

Back at my desk, I stare at my letter again. I mutter, "A few more weeks, Chris. You can do it." And I will. But as long as I'm at Career-Force, I will continue to do what I love. I will help people match skills to professions, and visit the vending machine in my spare time.

· · ·

WEEKS AFTER I have completed my internship, I bring several of my pastel drawings to Webster's bookstore. Sam welcomes me with open arms. "Hello my friend," he says. "You have been patient and your day has come!" He means that today is the day I am going to set up for my art show.

"Thanks Sam."

I go over to the empty walls that are filled with nail holes, put my paintings on a coffee table, and I pull up a chair so I can reach the high places. One by one, I grab my drawings and carefully hang them in a fashion I feel is appropriate. Remembering some material learned in art classes, I attempt to apply certain aesthetic principles, so that the arrangement will pop out, encouraging observers to look more closely.

One of the main reasons I want to showcase my work is to build a reputation, for exposure. And as seen at the Arts Fest, expo-sure leads to bigger venues, and greater chances of selling some things. To some degree, it is about making money.

But even if this is the only show I have, it is a self-esteem builder. It is so satisfying. In the past three years, I have seen that all my practice at Old Main has led to drastic improvements in the quality of my artwork. My eye is catching the tiny details, the power of color experimentation and linear acuity.

I struggle to maintain my balance when hanging my work, but I eventually succeed. Once I have jumped off the chair, I walk to the back of the room. I have some drawings at eye level, my Joe Paterno portraits, some above, just general football drawings, and some below, more portraits, one of which is of my angelic Mary Grace. When I finish examining the layout of my work, I conclude that everything is perfect.

Sam walks to the back of the room too, stands right next to me. He nods, I hope, in approval. I smirk. I can't help it. I mean I just can't wait for everyone to see this!

• • •

"**H**EY DR. Webber," I say over the phone the following day. "How are you doing?" When she replies, she is as animated as when I worked with her at CareerForce. Which would mean hardly at all. "Well. Hello Chris. What can I do for you?"

"I was just wondering if you'd like to bring some of the kids to an art exhibit this week. I'm displaying my artwork at Webster's bookstore. Somehow tie the trip to the vocational material in your curriculum."

She sighs. "I was actually just thinking about my plan for the day. You know the summer program is over, but I think Jane and Jerry would enjoy that. Do you think we could make the visit today?"

"Anytime today."

"Wonderful."

In the afternoon, Dr. Webber walks into the bookstore. In a pair of slacks and a different plaid, button-down shirt, she approaches me, greets me, and pats me on the back. "Good to see you, Chris."

"You too." I look past Dr. Webber, and see Jerry and Jane standing there. I am excited to see them, but, like many teens, they aren't enthusiastic about our reunion. Their shoulders sag, and their hellos are half-hearted. "Well," I continue. "Come in and I'll show you my stuff."

The bookstore is small, so the tour is brief, but I spend some time explaining my techniques and the process of painting a portrait. I do it in a way that is easy for Jerry and Jane to grasp, and explain to them that you can find jobs that allow you to use my techniques.

After I'm done, I let them look some more. I stand back, and just watch them. They seem very interested, and it really makes me feel good. Except for the day we visited Penn Tech, I rarely saw the students actively participate in the activities, so their positive reactions to my paintings are a welcome surprise.

When they finish observing everything, Jerry walks and Jane limps to the café, and they both buy drinks from Sam. Dr. Webber follows after them, thanks me, compliments me, and bids me farewell.

I don't receive any compliments the rest of the week, but this is fine. I know I'm a decent artist. It is nice to hear that people enjoy realism over the abstract, however I really don't need the affirmation. I'm content with my work, and that's what matters, right?

• • •

THE LAST night of my show, it dawns on me that I should invite Alex and Sam to my graduation. In talking to Sam before I left the bookstore, my trusted mentor said, "You know, I always wanted to father a son from start to finish. You've been that son, but now you're leaving. Now I have to find someone else." Alex has been a friend who always wanted a real father figure. It only makes sense to me that I introduce the two at the ceremony, so that both men might have their dreams fulfilled.

It also dawns on me that perhaps John would benefit from meeting my practicum supervisor, Mrs. Patterson. His negative feelings about teachers might change, if he sees that he can connect on a personal level with a professor, and live without fear of repercussions.

Excited, I spend the rest of the night making calls and presenting invitations. All of the invites accept, and, while it makes me very happy that they are coming, I get a little nervous, too. In a good way.

My final call is the most significant to me. I am again going to talk to Mary Grace. If she could make it to the graduation ceremony, she would make up for Michael's absence tenfold. What could be better than to have my dear angel present during my day of celebration? I think, *Nothing*, as I dial her number.

After three rings, I hear Mary Grace's voice. "Hello?" Man, is it a sweet voice!

"Hey Mary Grace. It's Chris."

"Oh, hi Chris. This is a surprise."

"I hope I'm not calling too late."

"No. Not yet. Getting ready to go to bed, but not yet." I imagine her sitting at the edge of her bed, delicately combing her long hair.

"I don't want to keep you, but I was just calling to see if you'd be interested in coming to my graduation tomorrow. Admission and seating is free." I think, *Please say yes. Please say yes.*

"Well. Thank you for asking, and I'd love to, but I can't promise anything." I hear her mattress squeak. "I mean . . . I don't know if I'll be called into work."

"Just thought I'd invite you. It would be great to see you again."

"I'll try," she says, yawning. "If I can, I need to get my rest, right?" I see her pulling back her covers, and pulling them up to her neck as she curls up beneath them, smiling.

"You are definitely right," I agree. "Sleep well." She hangs up the phone, and I start getting ready for bed.

● ● ●

WELL. IT'S finally here! Graduation day! Two in the afternoon, here, and am I ever having difficulty with my black gown! Actually, it's not so much the gown as it is the hood. The hood is like a window curtain, only the dark blue satin fabric is supposed to drape around my shoulders, and the light blue stripes along the edges are supposed to bunch up at the back. It has to be folded properly. The directions in the gown packet I purchased a while back make it look so easy. False advertising, in my opinion. My hood looks nothing like the picture.

What makes it worse, is the fact that I am running out of time. I am in line, waiting my turn to get my picture taken with my family at the Nittany Lion Shrine, the stone statue of Penn State's mascot. The people ahead of me are finishing up with their photo shoots relatively fast, and I am desperately asking anyone around me to help out. I can tell one or two families are getting agitated; some others are getting a kick out of my troubles. But no one seems to know how to fold the hood. After several failed attempts, I tell those people behind me to go on ahead. And after another series of faulty folding, my parents and grandparents agree that my back will be out of sight and we will worry about my appearance later.

The Lion Shrine is a beautiful sculpture, a gift given by a graduating class years ago, I think. It is one of the most visited tourist attractions on campus throughout the year, primarily during football season, but also on graduation day. Having a photo at this site on this triumphant day will bring back fond memories in the future, I'm sure.

I know that I will look back and recall the evenings I stopped walking along the brick sidewalk just to stand before the shining landmark, one hand on my hip, to admire the craftsmanship, to motivate myself to represent my university well, and to remind myself that God made me a Nittany Lion for a reason.

When all of my family have climbed and reached the peak of the mulch-strewn mound surrounding the shrine, we huddle close together as someone gladly takes our picture for us. To my right, my grandmother laughs hard, says, "Can you believe you've done it?" and makes sure my cap is on correctly, pushing my tassel aside so it isn't blocking my face. To my left, my grandpa is grinning, says, "What do ya' say, buddy? You ready?" and lovingly squeezes me. The camera flashes three times, and the lady taking the picture says, "Beautiful!"

After I have finished posing with Grandma and Grandpa, my father and I stand right next to the lion and hug each other. Grandpa takes several shots. It is extremely windy, my gown isn't deflecting it at all, and my hood is flailing, so Dad and I descend the mound, step around one of the lights that makes the famous cat glow at night, and walk to the car intent on going to the Performing Arts Building, where the graduation ceremony will take place.

I have to be there at three, and I should make it on time.

• • •

I ARRIVE AT the Performing Arts Building at three, exactly. My chest progressively pounds as I walk towards the entrance, my heartbeat increasing because I'm filled with emotion. I'm feeling eager, nervous, proud, and, I admit, even vulnerable. You name it; I'm feeling it. Climbing the stairs, I see other students in their gowns and caps, with their hoods improperly folded as well, and it eases my concerns about my attire.

Upon entering the building, I examine the layout of the foyer, the maroon carpeting, the soft maroon benches along the walls, and the table in the center, where I have to get my name tag with my college and major printed on it. The doors to the auditorium are still closed, and, for the most part, except for a beautifully decorated conifer in the corner, the area is empty. The stillness and the beautiful décor makes me feel warm on the inside, slows my heartbeat some.

I walk up to the table lined in black, ruffled cloth and ask one of the three ushers in classy tuxedos to give me my name tag. The lady usher marks my name on the list, and kindly tells me not to lose the card because I'll have to hand it in before I go on stage. As I walk away from the table, I think, *Well, that was easy enough. Relax, Chris.* And my heartbeat becomes a slow patter.

Between observing the building and speaking with the ushers, I was so caught up in the moment, feeling so warm, that I didn't realize how many graduates and family members had come in. They are still coming through the front doors. Most of the graduates appear to be as emotional as I am, excited about graduating, but uncertain about ceremony protocol.

One thing they all are doing is repositioning gowns and hoods. Husbands are helping graduating wives. Wives are helping graduating husbands. Parents are helping their graduating sons and daughters. And Grandparents are helping graduating grandchildren.

I am intrigued by how differently people of other ethnic backgrounds are prepping themselves here. From what I've seen, the Asians are doing so in a reserved and thorough manner. The Africans seem to be the happiest, making small talk about the gowns. The African Americans are the most verbal, laughing loudly at their dressing difficulties. And the Whites appear to be satisfied with whatever works, somewhat indifferent about the whole thing.

JOSHUA HOLMES

My Grandparents and Parents are happily walking in my direction to help me prep. Only this time, an assistant who has helped graduates tidy up in the past is walking by their side to move the process forward more quickly, and, most importantly, make me look good. I have to say, that, after my tie is pulled tight, my gown is zipped up, my hood is in place, and my cap is on, I feel awesome.

Not long after the director has finished cleaning me up, and my family takes more pictures, do the other ushers open the doors to the auditorium, and point the graduates to separate doors, to find their colleges and stand in the assigned area until further notice. Before I do so, I glance back at my family, and see that everyone I invited, except for Michael and Linda, is here. Content, I go and find my college, The College of Education, by looking at the colors on the hood, and stand there with several students I have never seen or heard before.

I stand for a long time. I even talk to some of the students.

• • •

A FUNNY, OLDER gentleman in full, purple satin garb interrupts all the students in conversation. "We're starting soon, everyone. Let me look at your hoods!" He goes from person to person, turns the decorative pieces around when necessary, and gives us a history lesson on the origin of the dress. I hear him say "Way back in the day . . ." several times before we all line up.

Golden posts with vinyl ribbons are positioned so that I and my fellow graduates must march single file, as we all make our way into the auditorium, and descend the sloping walkway. The floor is carpeted maroon, like in the foyer, and the walls are colored a light pink. Large cup-like, golden lights are evenly placed on an extended parapet, the place more formal than anything I've seen.

And the place is packed; let me tell you. I'm taken aback. Considering no one needed tickets to attend, I thought the place would almost be empty. Man was I wrong. Not only are the ground seats filled, but the seats in the balcony are, as well. I can't help but admire the carved, white concrete colonnades that support the balcony, too.

As I reach my reserved row of seats, I wait until the funny man instructs me to start towards my seat. I feel awkward walking in front of the already seated audience. This whole scene feels bigger than life. I accomplished a lot, yes, but all of this attention? I don't know. I'm a simple guy who doesn't like to receive a lot of public notice. "Holy Crap," I mutter. "This is crazy."

• • •

THE MAN who presents the commencement speech is a revered dean with numerous credentials President Graham Spanier, among others, finds valuable. The credentials mean nothing to me. He gives a crazy dialogue about climate change, the slow demise of human existence, and the graduates' role in making the general public aware of it. Apparently, he believes, we, "having achieved a level of education many have not," have a responsibility to go out into the world and promote change. A talk about climate change at a graduation ceremony? I don't know what the President was thinking!

After sitting almost forty-five minutes through the depressing dialogue, and thirty more minutes through the procession of the doctoral candidates, watching their professors hood their students, and the dean handing them their diplomas, the master's students in my row are instructed to stand and walk out of the auditorium, out to the area where I stood previously, to go to the back stairwell leading to the curtained platform, and, finally, to hand my name card into a woman who is responsible for telling me when to walk onstage.

As I wait, I think back to earlier in the day, the few moments just prior to my departure from the lobby, when I saw John conversing with Mrs. Patterson, no sign of animosity towards my professor, no indication in his face that his childhood was making it difficult to socialize with the lady I initially had difficulties with. She nodded her head repeatedly, smiled, and gazed at him deeply, her eyes full of empathy. Perhaps her sensitivity had helped him come to a realization that he could overcome his past.

And, right behind John and Mrs. Patterson, I saw Sam and Alex laughing with one another; the old man patting my friend on the back, encouraging him, I'm sure. Alex's forehead was plastered in creases, fissures of happiness, to my delight. Sam had his dreads neatly pulled back into a ponytail of sorts, his minimal attempt at formality. I felt good seeing two people so different so satisfied with each other's company at an event honoring my achievement.

Back in the present, I hear a "psssst." I look behind me, at the woman who I handed my name card to. "It's your turn. Start walking." This is the moment I've been waiting for, for two long years. I take a deep breath, soak up the moment, and commit it to memory. In my long gown, I glide onto the stage and do as the Doctoral students did, shake hands with the president, and the deans. Over the speakers, I hear my name and major called out. *Finally!* I think. *It is over!* I look out into the crowd, watching for my family and friends.

I spot them all half way across the platform. Talk about an absolute, a truth no one can dispute. Not Plato. Not Aristotle. Not anyone! When I see my Parents and Grandparents, Sam, John, Alex, and my angel Mary Grace, the view is as vivid as any I would see in a dream during a seizure. Only this is not a dream. And I am definitely not having a Grand Mal.

THE END

ACKNOWLEDGMENTS

Thanks to God, my Parents, and Grandparents